Discordant Pandemic Narratives in the U.S.

Discordant Pandemic Narratives in the U.S.

Edited by Shing-Ling S. Chen and Nicole Allaire

LEXINGTON BOOKS
Lanham • Boulder • New York • London

Published by Lexington Books
An imprint of The Rowman & Littlefield Publishing Group, Inc.
4501 Forbes Boulevard, Suite 200, Lanham, Maryland 20706
www.rowman.com

6 Tinworth Street, London SE11 5AL, United Kingdom

British Library Cataloguing in Publication Information Available

Library of Congress Cataloging-in-Publication Data Available

ISBN 978-1-7936-5533-2 (cloth: alk. paper)
ISBN 978-1-7936-5534-9 (electronic)

Dedicated to

Carl J. Couch

(1925–1994)

The Study of Humanity for Humanity

Contents

Introduction

Discordant Narratives and Social Chaos

Shing-Ling S. Chen

Coronavirus disease 2019 (COVID-19) is a highly contagious and severe acute respiratory disease which was first identified in China in December 2019. The disease has since spread around the world as an ongoing pandemic. So far the disease has caused more than five million deaths worldwide.

The United States is the country with the highest number of deaths caused by COVID-19, having more than 850,000 Americans who died of COVID-19. Despite the wealth of resources and advancement in technologies, the U.S. failed to respond to the pandemic effectively and efficiently. In fact, the U.S. pandemic responses have been chaotic from the start, which, as the authors in this volume would argue, stems from the discordant pandemic narratives in the U.S.

Unlike Germany, Taiwan, or New Zealand, where there was a united national front combating COVID-19, the pandemic narratives in the U.S. were discordant. Narratives, structures of storytelling, are believed to be able to help groups and individuals make sense of the environment and ease the nerves in an uncertain time (Maines, 2001). However, the U.S. pandemic narratives which embodied many conflicting structures failed to provide guidance for groups and individuals to construct a clear understanding of the pandemic or a consistent measure to combat the disease.

The discordant narratives originated in the Situation Room in the White House among members of the White House Coronavirus Task Force, which then spilled over into the Task Force's daily briefings, creating conflicting narratives between then President Donald Trump and Dr. Anthony Fauci, a key figure on the Task Force, on issues regarding shelter-in-place, masks, anti-malaria drugs, etc. The conflicting views of Trump and Fauci confused the American public, at a critical time when clear guidance was needed.

On the state level, facing a national pandemic, governors looked to Trump for leadership; however, Trump told the governors that they were on their own, as Trump saw himself not as a national leader, but merely as a sideline supporter, when combating the pandemic. It was a dire circumstance for governors, as most of the governors had no experience in dealing with such a severe pandemic as COVID-19. Governors had many complaints about the lack of federal guidance and help. One of the complaints was the competition from the federal government for medical supplies amid a shortage, as the federal government worked to increase its own stockpile.

In business, companies made their own safety rules as the federal government stood aside. Unsafe rules were implemented, workers went to work fearing for their lives. Conflicting practices were found in industries due to free-wheeling interpretations of government recommendations. Inconsistent practices led to outbreaks in meatpacking plants, long-term care facilities, etc.

In addition, there was discordance among citizens in the U.S. Amid the pandemic and the Centers for Disease Control and Prevention (CDC) warnings against travel, and social gathering, tens of thousands of Americans continued to travel nationally and internationally, go on vacations, and host large social gatherings and church services.

On the individual level, discordant practices were omnipresent. A clear example was masking. Many who denied the pandemic followed the belief of individualism, argued that masking violated body autonomy, and hence, refused to mask. Others who were concerned about self-wellbeing, as well as public health, masked consistently.

Due to the discordant narratives and chaotic responses, the death toll of COVID-19 stacked up quickly in the U.S. A fatality count equal to two Vietnam Wars was recorded in just two months after the pandemic outbreak in January 2020. By October 2020, more than a quarter-million lives had been lost. By February 2021, more than half a million lives were lost in the U.S. due to the pandemic.

The COVID-19 pandemic, a historical catastrophe, with such a high death toll, clearly calls for a careful examination of the discordant narratives that embodied the chaos, tensions, and conflicts in the U.S. pandemic responses. Authors in this volume address the various forms of discordance found in pandemic narratives in the U.S. The purpose of the volume is to address the theoretical significance, as well as the social, cultural, and political implications of the pandemic discordance.

In "Economy vs. Public Health: Discordant Leadership Narratives in the Pandemic," Shing-Ling S. Chen and Zanetta Miller examine the forms of discordance found in the leadership of President Trump and President Biden in their efforts of combating the COVID-19 pandemic. They argue that Trump's insistence on the stability and wellbeing of the economy stipulated his inaction on the pandemic in the early months, as well as his public conflict with Fauci, politicizing the CDC, and his free-rein leadership style that created chaos on both the national level and the state level. Trump's successor, Biden, adopted the leadership style called for in crisis communication to quickly combat the pandemic. However, Biden faced much opposition and resistance.

In "Mandates vs. No Mandates: Communitarianism and Libertarianism in the Pandemic," Melissa L. Beall and Shing-Ling S. Chen look into two important mandates during the pandemic—mask mandates and vaccine mandates—and the significant oppositions the mandates created. They indicate the need to adopt communitarianism, instead of libertarianism when addressing a highly contagious disease. In addition, by examining the mandates and their resistances, Beall and Chen expand the discussion of leadership in crisis communication, by indicating the need to construct a solidary relationship in a group when a leader adopts the needed autocratic leadership in a crisis situation. The solidary relationship created, they argue, would not only ease the opposition but also expedite the accomplishment of the social objective in a crisis situation.

In "Religious Freedom vs. Public Health: Discordant Legal Narratives in the Pandemic," Juliet Dee highlights the conflicts between public health officials and religious leaders regarding social distancing requirements and lockdown orders in the pandemic where religious leaders filed lawsuits against their state governments. Dee analyzed the legal arguments in cases where judges balanced the conflicting claims of free exercise of religion as well as freedom of assembly, and the right of local, state, and federal officials to enforce regulations to protect public health. Dee found that judges applied the *ad hoc balancing theory* of First Amendment law in deciding cases, resulting in discordant court decisions.

Rachel Kaplan, in "Domestic Disjointed Narratives of the Pandemic: The Critical Early Months," illustrates the lack of a global narrative in the U.S. when addressing the COVID-19 pandemic in the early months of 2020. Kaplan analyzes the shifting frames of the pandemic from a naive perception of the disease as a problem of the "other," to an erroneous prediction that COVID-19 would bring economic prosperity to the U.S., as manufacturing industries would re-shore due to the illness, in January 2020, to President Trump's inaccurate optimism that the virus would disappear as the temperatures rose, in early March 2020. The author then notes that by mid-March, the alarms sounded as schools began to close due to the widespread illness; and by the end of April 2020, the virus claimed more American lives than the

Vietnam War. The analysis demonstrates the lack of a global understanding of a highly contagious disease that could easily spread worldwide. The lack of a global understanding, coupled with an erroneous domestic narrative, led the administration to essentially do nothing in the critical early months of the pandemic, which subsequently resulted in tens of thousands of unnecessary, preventable, deaths and sufferings. Kaplan's chapter highlights the importance of the notion of space, a cornerstone in communication research.

In "Historical vs. Ahistorical Narratives of the Pandemic: The Discordant Rhetoric of Our Unprecedented Times, " John J. Rief argues that there was a lack of historical narratives when the U.S. media reported the COVID-19 pandemic, as the media presented a pernicious divide between our current pandemic moment and our historical experiences. Media coverage of the pandemic was thoroughly saturated by the claim that our times are "unprecedented." By doing so, the media rendered our history unavailable as a resource to engage this pandemic critically. Rief argues that the media adopted an ahistorical narrative to construct our times as unprecedented, which ultimately undermines sense-making and decision-making, leaving us with no ground upon which to understand our context and respond to it. Rief lays out a more informative historical narrative structure that situates COVID-19 in a historical context of contagious diseases in the U.S. and worldwide and calls for adopting a historical narrative to understand the current pandemic as well as to construct courses of action. Rief's chapter features the importance of the notion of time in communication research.

Tyler Welsh, R. Tyler Spradley, and Elizabeth Spradley in "Discordant Rhetorical Responses: Crisis Communication in Sports Organizations in the Covid-19 Pandemic" analyzed how professional sports responded to the COVID-19 pandemic. Their analysis serves to illustrate the different narratives that sports administrators adopted to respond to the pandemic, and evaluate the different practices and impacts as an outcome. Welsh, R. Spradley, and E. Spradley studied the National Football League (NFL) and the National Basketball Association (NBA), utilizing Kenneth Burke's concept of *representative anecdotes* to examine how these two organizations attempted to handle the disease safely while remaining operational. They report that while the NBA constructed a quarantined "bubble" that allowed games to continue, the NFL left decisions open for individual franchises to make and implement, even though franchises lacked experience in handling such a large-scale crisis. They point out the narrative adopted by the NFL did reduce the economic impact of the pandemic on the league. They then indicate how these discordant leadership narratives in professional sports resembled the discordant leadership narratives found in the Trump administration, unlike the administrations of other countries such as Germany and New Zealand. With their analysis, one can ascertain the merit of Trump's decision to let governors battle the pandemic was to reduce the negative impacts of the pandemic on the economy, as the NFL illustrated.

In "Misinformation, Scandalization, and the *Trump Show*: Audience Responses to President Trump's Pandemic Narrative," Kristjan Kikerpill set out to find out how the audience perceived Trump's statements, in two subsequent media interviews, after he had made two erroneous suggestions to combat the coronavirus—by injecting bleach and using light "inside the body." Kikerpill wonders if the audience perceived Trump's statements as information which one would expect from a head of state in crisis communication, or if the audience perceived Trump's utterances as dark entertainment. Kikerpill reports that Trump's supporters who were attracted to Trump's cult of personality viciously defended Trump, while those who opposed Trump posted mockery comments where they viewed Trump's comments as entertainment. Kikerpill indicates that the polarized groups did not see Trump's statements as factual or to-the-point, needed in crisis communication. Kikerpill also cautions that the media's scandalization of President Trump's misinformation, in search of high TV ratings, might have harmed the general populace in times of crisis.

Stephen D. Caldes, Zach Justus, and Jennifer A. Malkowski, in "Manufacturing Disinformation: The Story of *Plandemic*," illustrate the techniques used to construct a piece of convincing disinformation, deliberately deceptive and computational propaganda, *Plandemic*. *Plandemic,* a twenty-six-minute viral video, released in May 2020, presents a conspiracy narrative, aimed at provoking discordance and undermining U.S. COVID-19 responses. Caldes, Justus, and Malkowski analyzed the video to demonstrate how a host of false and misleading claims were weaved into a convincing narrative. By analyzing the storytelling techniques used in *Plandemic*, they illustrate how the video was used to mobilize conspiracy theorists, undermine the public health agenda, and introduce uncertainty into the public.

The objective of the volume is twofold: to use the pandemic discordance to illustrate various theories that inform the analyses, as well as to use the theories to provide a deeper understanding of the pandemic discordance in social, cultural, and political contexts. The ultimate goal of this volume is to help groups and individuals understand just what went wrong in the U.S. pandemic responses, which resulted in the highest death toll in the world.

REFERENCE

Maines, D. (2001). *The faultline of consciousness: A view of interactionism in sociology*. Milton Park, UK: Routledge.

Chapter One

Economy vs. Public Health

Discordant Leadership Narratives in the Pandemic

Shing-Ling S. Chen and Zanetta Miller

In 2020, during the COVID-19 pandemic, former President Donald Trump's leadership in the U.S. garnished much criticism. Many attributed the chaotic pandemic responses in the U.S. to issues of his leadership. This chapter utilizes the literature in narrative research in the field of sociology, as well as leadership studies in the field of management, to provide an analysis of Trump's leadership responding to the pandemic in 2020. The purposes of the analysis are to provide a fine-grained view and assessment of many issues raised regarding Trump's leadership.

Sociologist Carl Couch (1987) had noted the importance to compare and contrast similar activities of individuals in different sets of social interactions in order to provide a thorough understanding of issues examined. Hence, to better understand the social forms of Trump's activities, some comparisons with the activities of Trump's successor, President Joe Biden, are used. The contrast and comparison serves to highlight the forms of Trump's activities as well as the alternative forms of actions which could have been taken.

To analyze a wide array of actions by Trump and those by Biden, this essay utilizes the analytical schemes established in narrative research (Maines, 2001) to illustrate the persistent values and beliefs adhered to by each president, and the related actions adopted, in their responses to the COVID-19 pandemic. According to David Maines (2001), narrative refers to cultural paradigms or structures of group life, and story refers to anything reported that contains a plot. Maines (2001) asserts, "Narrative structures are cultural frames and ideologies that prefigure some stories insofar as group beliefs and values contain already-articulated plots" (p. 206). Using narrative structures and stories as guidelines, the following discussion illustrates the dominant paradigms or structures of Trump's and Biden's COVID-19 responses, the narratives, as well as the actions adopted by the respective administrations, the stories, to support the dominant narrative.

TRUMP'S ECONOMY NARRATIVE

Throughout 2020, then President Donald Trump adhered to the economy as his priority when handling the coronavirus, as he had wagered his re-election on the economy. In January 2020, when Trump was informed by his advisers about the seriousness of the coronavirus, and the need for aggressive action, Trump repeatedly played down the seriousness of the situation. Lipton and associates indicate,

> Even after Mr. Azar [U.S. Secretary of Health and Human Services] first briefed him about the potential seriousness of the virus during a phone call on Jan. 18 while the president was at his Mar-a-Lago resort in Florida, Mr. Trump projected confidence that it would be a passing problem. (Lipton et al., 2020, para. 79)

When asked by the media about what actions to take regarding the coronavirus, Trump assured the media that "We have it totally under control," and "It's going to be just fine," in an interview a few days later [after Jan. 18] while attending the World Economic Forum in Switzerland (Lipton et al., 2020, para. 80).

It was also reported that when making decisions regarding the pandemic, instead of relying on the recommendations of the health experts, Trump paid close attention to the stock market. Trump was concerned that any action in combating the coronavirus would cause a stock market decline or economic slowdown which would then hinder his re-election effort. It was reported that he would seek advice from prominent investors who recommended Trump not to issue a lockdown and keep the economy open. Lipton and associates quote some of Trump's speeches in April 2020, e.g., "Everybody [prominent investors] questioned it for a while, not everybody, but a good portion questioned it"; "They said, let's keep it open. Let's ride it" (Lipton et al., 2020, para. 100).

However, it was clear in late February 2020, that schools and businesses were hotspots of the virus. Trump finally agreed to issue social distancing guidelines nationwide in mid-March, which brought much of the economy to a halt. To some of his associates Trump was described as "shell-shocked and deflated" and "subdued" and "baffled" as he had to issue a call that disrupted much of the economy, which Trump "had wagered his re-election on and was suddenly in shambles" (Lipton et al., 2020, para. 12).

In May 2020, after the Trump administration had presented the governors with the broad guidelines for reopening, it was reported that the White House pressured governors to reopen businesses as soon as possible. Mayor Francis Suarez of Miami stated, "It was all predicated on reduction, open, reduction, open more, reduction, open. . . . There was never what happens if there is an increase after you reopen?" (Shear, Weiland, Lipton, Haberman, & Sanger, 2020, para. 96). Trump's concern for the economy permeated throughout his actions in combating the pandemic in 2020.

Examining the activities of the Trump administration over time, Trump's adherence to the economy, instead of public health, was not a simple misjudgment, but a consistent paradigm that his administration adhered to in the pandemic. Shear and associates explain,

> Mr. Trump's bet that the crisis would fade away proved wrong. But an examination of the shift in April and its aftermath shows that the approach he embraced was not just a misjudgment. Instead, it was a deliberate strategy that he would stick doggedly to as evidence mounted that, in the absence of strong leadership from the White House, the virus would continue to infect and kill large numbers of Americans. (Shear et al., 2020, para. 11)

To apply Maines's narrative analytical scheme (2001), Trump's firm value and belief in safeguarding the security of the economy, due to the concern of his re-election, constitute the narrative of his leadership. The following discussion reports an array of actions adopted by his administration to support Trump's economy narrative. These actions are considered as stories that illuminate Trump's economy narrative structure.

A Divided Task Force: Trump vs. Fauci

The first case of COVID-19 was found in Washington State on January 20, 2020. By the end of January 2020, the White House Coronavirus Task Force was established. The task force, situated in the United States Department of State in the Trump administration, coordinated and oversaw the administration's efforts to mitigate the COVID-19 pandemic in the U.S. The task force was initially chaired by Alex Azar, Secretary of Health and Human Services, when it was established in January 2020. In February 2020, U.S. vice president Mike Pence became the chair of the task force.

The task force live-streamed press briefings for updates and policies. In March 2020, the White House held the task force press briefings daily. Trump was present in the press briefings and he dominated the discussions as he believed the briefings provided him good public perceptions. At the daily press briefings, it was noted,

> Mr. Trump is typically joined at his briefings by top medical advisers, including Dr. Fauci and Dr. Deborah L. Birx, his coronavirus coordinator. But the president does most of the talking and has told several advisers that the briefings give him free airtime and good ratings. (Crowley, Thomas, & Haberman, 2020, para. 19)

However, in April, there was a reduced frequency of the task force briefings, when the administration set its priority on the economy and reopening. In late April 2020, there was no briefing held. By October 2020, the number of task force meetings had diminished.

The task force was not only made up of health officials but also experts in various fields, such as economy, politics, labor force, etc. Hence, without having public health as a pivot, disagreements among members of the task force arose. Concerns about public health often clashed with the concerns about the economy. It was reported that the debates over whether to adhere to Trump's economy narrative or to shut down much of the country, which would bring the economy to a halt, were fierce (Shear et al., 2020). The conflict between the economic narrative and the public health narrative in the task force also played out in public in the conflicting messages uttered by Trump and those by Dr. Anthony Fauci.

Fauci is a renowned infectious disease expert in the U.S., and "is a leading member of the White House's coronavirus task force and the director of the National Institute of Allergy and Infectious Diseases, making him a trusted, and popular, voice as the U.S. deals with a deadly pandemic" (Behrmann & Santucci, 2020, para. 2). Trump's insistence on the economy clashed with Fauci's priority on public health on numerous occasions.

In February 2020, at a political rally, Trump downplayed the seriousness of the coronavirus and asserted that the coronavirus would be gone by April 2020, when the weather became warmer (Subramanian, Behrmann, & Jackson, 2020). Fauci, on the other hand, indicated that scientists did not know how the coronavirus would impact society, hence, he disagreed with Trump, and stated, "So we would think it would be a stretch to assume that it's going to disappear with the warm weather. We don't know that. It's completely unknown" (CBS News, 2020, para. 34).

In March 2020, at a White House coronavirus press briefing, Trump boasted that hydroxychloroquine, a drug to treat malaria, as a "game-changer" in treating COVID-19, implying a quick fix was in sight, and everything, including the economy, would be back to normal. Speaking after Trump, Fauci downplayed the effects of the drug as based on "anecdotal evidence"

(Behrmann & Santucci, 2020, para. 19). Then, Trump, standing behind Fauci, stepped forward to claim: "We'll see. We're going to know soon" (Behrmann & Santucci, 2020, para. 20). When later being asked about his reactions to Trump's untruthful statements, Fauci stated, "But I can't jump in front of the microphone and push him [Trump] down" (Cohen, 2020, para. 15).

In April 2020, the disagreement on hydroxychloroquine between Trump and Fauci continued. At the news briefing on Sunday, April 5, 2020, Trump continued to recommend the anti-malaria drug as an effective drug against the coronavirus and called for widely administering the drug. Trump acknowledged that he was speaking on gut instinct and he had no expertise on the subject (Crowley et al., 2020). However, Trump was very confident about the outlook of the anti-malaria drug. Crowley and associates report on this issue,

> Saying that the drug is "being tested now," Mr. Trump said that "there are some very strong, powerful signs" of its potential, although health experts say that the data is extremely limited and that more study of the drug's effectiveness against the coronavirus is needed. (Crowley et al., 2020, para. 5)

Fauci, standing alongside Trump at the news briefing, who had been skeptical about the drug's potential, had declined to endorse Trump's claim about the effectiveness of hydroxychloroquine. Therefore, "when a reporter at Sunday's briefing asked Dr. Anthony S. Fauci, the director of the National Institute of Allergy and Infectious Diseases, to weigh in on the subject [hydroxychloroquine], Mr. Trump stopped him [Fauci] from answering" (Cowley, Thomas, & Haberman, 2020, para. 9). Trump publicly silenced Fauci, knowing Fauci would not support his claim about hydroxychloroquine.

To show his dismay of Fauci, Trump retweeted a post by DeAnna Lorraine, a former congressional candidate, which called for firing Fauci:

> "Fauci is now saying that had Trump listened to the medical experts earlier he could've saved more lives. Fauci was telling people on February 29th that there was nothing to worry about and it posed no threat to the US public at large. Time to #FireFauci," former congressional candidate DeAnna Lorraine wrote on Twitter. (Orr & Levine, 2020, para. 3)

In addition, in May 2020, Trump blocked Fauci from testifying about the coronavirus response before the Appropriation Committee in the House of Representatives. Trump did not wish to have Fauci appear in front of the Democratic-controlled House, unfriendly to Trump (Emma & Cook, 2020). Trump told the reporters, "The House is a setup. . . . The House is a bunch of Trump haters. They put every Trump hater on the committee" (Page, 2020, para. 10). Instead, Trump had Fauci testify in the Republican-led Senate, friendly to Trump, and asserted that Fauci "will be testifying in front of the Senate, and looks forward to doing that" (para. 10).

In his testimony in the Senate, Fauci contradicted Trump's plans to ease stay-at-home restrictions and to have school openings, as well as Trump's claim that the virus might disappear without a vaccine. Page (2020) reports,

> Anthony Fauci, the top infectious-disease expert at the National Institutes of Health, works for President Donald Trump, of course. But with a measured tone in a grave voice and a distinctive Brooklyn accent, Fauci effectively undercut the message that his boss had championed the day before about how to respond to COVID-19. Trump was impatient, quick to claim success, and eager to have the country begin reopening. Fauci counseled patience, saying the medical realities mean the nation isn't ready to reopen and that doing it too early would carry a deadly cost. (para. 2)

By doing so, what the country witnessed was a showdown between the president and his medical adviser. To the public, "it was the president vs. the doctor, the commander-in-chief in the Rose Garden on Monday [May 11, 2020] and the nation's most trusted doctor in a Senate hearing room on Tuesday [May 12, 2020]" (Page, 2020, para. 1). According to a poll conducted by CBS News, after Fauci's Senate testimony, it showed that Fauci was trusted by most and viewed favorably by a three to one margin—with 62 percent trusting and 38 percent not trusting Fauci, as well as 46 percent viewing Fauci favorably and 14 percent unfavorably (Khanna & Backus, 2020).

In early July 2020, it was reported that the Trump administration had "strayed from the advice of many of its scientists and public health experts" and "sidelined Fauci, scuttled some of his planned TV appearances, and largely kept him out of the Oval Office for more than a month" (Abutaleb, Dawsey, & McGinley, 2020, para. 2). Fauci confirmed that he had not briefed Trump for more than two months despite the pandemic resurgence (Wu, 2020). Further, Trump solicited support from users on Twitter about sidelining Fauci. He shared a post by Chuck Woolery, a TV show host, claiming that doctors and the CDC are lying. Woolery (2020) tweets, "The most outrageous lies are the ones about Covid 19. Everyone is lying. The CDC, Media, Democrats, our Doctors, not all but most, that we are told to trust." Trump also shared another tweet post that slammed Fauci: "So based on Dr. Fauci and the Democrats, I will need an ID card to go shopping but not to vote?" (Young, 2020).

Over the course of months working for Trump, "[Fauci] was accused of inventing the virus and of being part of a secret cabal with Bill Gates and George Soros to profit from vaccines. His family received death threats" (McNeil, 2002, para. 3). Fauci was eventually banished from public view due to his grim assessment of the pandemic. The discordance between Trump and Fauci illustrates Trump's denial of the pandemic, rejection of science, and ignoring the opinions of health experts, which were done due to preserving his economic narrative.

Politicizing the CDC

Knowing that the CDC, the highest authority in disease and health information in the country, may have been incongruent with Trump's economic narrative in managing the pandemic, the Trump administration interfered with the agency's work. Matt Pottinger, the deputy national security adviser, noted Trump's efforts in politicizing the health institutions to be in accordance with his economic narrative. In fact, "the CDC and FDA became captive agencies of the propaganda wing of the Trump administration" (*PBS*, 2020, para. 21).

Kyle McGowan, a former chief of staff at the CDC, and his deputy, Amanda Campbell, pointed out that during the 2020 coronavirus pandemic what they witnessed was "Washington's dismissal of science, the White House's slow suffocation of the agency's voice, the meddling in its messages and the siphoning of its budget" (Weiland, 2021a, para. 2). With the White House fixated on the economic implications of public health, "[the] White House insisted on reviewing—and often softening—the CDC's closely guarded coronavirus guidance documents . . . " (Weiland, 2021a, para. 10). There were many incidences where the Trump administration stifled the CDC. One notable instance was that the CDC had to negotiate with the Trump administration over social distancing guidelines for restaurants. The White House had complained that spacing recommendations by the CDC would be too onerous for businesses to enforce. Due to the concern of the economic viability of the restaurant industry, the CDC had to compromise by recommending social distancing without a reference to the six-foot measurement (Weiland, 2021a). Kyle McGowan told of another notable incidence:

> In the spring [2020], the CDC published an app that allowed Americans to screen themselves for symptoms of Covid-19. But the Trump administration decided to develop a similar tool with Apple. White House officials then demanded that the CDC wipe its app off its website. (Weiland, 2021a, para. 21)

Reacting to the interference that the Trump administration had on the operations of the CDC, McGowan said, "'Every time that the science clashed with the messaging, messaging won" (Weiland, 2021a, para. 20).

A notable incident of the Trump administration's meddling with the work of the CDC involved the agency's recommendation of mask-wearing. The CDC had drafted a sweeping order in September 2020, requiring all passengers and employees to wear masks on all forms of transportations in the U.S., but the order was blocked by the White House. Kaplan (2020) reported,

> The order would have been the toughest federal mandate to date aimed at curbing the spread of the coronavirus, which continues to infect more than 40,000 Americans a day. The officials said that it was drafted under the agency's "quarantine powers" and that it had the support of the secretary of health and human services, Alex M. Azar II, but the White House Coronavirus Task Force, led by Vice President Mike Pence, declined to even discuss it. (para. 2)

Not only with issues of social distancing in restaurants and the mask mandate, it was also noted that "political appointees at the White House and the Department of Health and Human Services have also been involved in rewriting the agency's guidelines on reopening schools and testing for the virus, bypassing the agency's scientists" (Kaplan, 2020, para. 9).

On July 8, 2020, the CDC published its recommendations detailing the risks of school reopening and the steps that districts had to take to minimize those risks (CDC, 2020). Always concerned with the economy, Trump quickly criticized the recommendations as "very tough and expensive" (*New York Times*, 2020). Two weeks later, a new set of CDC recommendations were published, which downplayed the potential health risks stated in the original recommendations. Instead, what the public saw was a blaring call to reopen schools, with the original recommendations being compromised by the White House administration:

> The top U.S. public health agency issued a full-throated call to reopen schools in a package of new "resources and tools" posted on its website Thursday night that opened with a statement that sounded more like a political speech than a scientific document, listing numerous benefits for children of being in school and downplaying the potential health risks. (*New York Times*, 2020, July 24, para. 1)

In July 2020, to deprive the CDC of the control of coronavirus data, the White House ordered hospitals to send all patient information to a central database in Washington beginning on July 8, bypassing the CDC where the hospitals had sent their patient information (Stolberg, 2020). Such an order "has alarmed health experts who fear the data will be politicized or withheld from the public" (para. 1). White House officials said that the change served to streamline data gathering. However, the information received by the White House would not be open to the public. By not making the information open to the public, such change affected the work of researchers and health officials who had relied on the CDC for data for research and decision making. Jen Kates, the director of global health and H.I.V. policy with the nonpartisan Kaiser Family Foundation, commented that what was affected was not the researchers and health officials but "access for reporters, access for the public to try to better understand what is happening with the outbreak" (Stolberg, 2020, para. 4).

The Trump administration had long been criticized by public health experts for politicizing the CDC. Such a change further intensified the politicizing concerns and cast doubts on the Trump administration in withholding important public health information. In addition, by depriving the CDC of important pandemic data, some health experts questioned how the CDC was to perform its work. Dr. Nicole Lurie, as assistant secretary under the former President Barack Obama administration, asserted, "Centralizing control of all data under the umbrella of an inherently political apparatus is dangerous and breeds distrust. . . . It appears to cut off the ability of agencies like CDC to do its basic job" (Stolberg, 2020, para. 10).

Depriving the CDC of access to the pandemic data was believed to be an important indicator of the Trump administration politicizing the agency. Florida Representative Donna Shalala who served as the health secretary in the Bill Clinton administration, stated, "Only the CDC has the expertise to collect data," and "I think any move to take responsibility away from the people who have the expertise is politicizing" (para. 22).

Inaction and Denial

In January 2020, Trump was aware that the U.S. had a problem with the coronavirus when the U.S. experienced its first coronavirus infections and was warned by medical experts to expect the outbreak to spread in the country. On January 30, 2020, the World Health Organization declared a global health emergency. But Trump continued to ignore the urgent requests from his medical advisers to issue a national stay-at-home order and do more to control the disease.

Trump dismissed the coronavirus threat from January to mid-March, thinking of the threat "as a small number of U.S. cases that were under 'control' and would fall to zero by April" (Woodward & Yen, 2020, para. 20). On February 10, 2020, Trump stated that "we're in great shape . . . we have 12 cases" and he told Fox Business that "in April, supposedly, it dies with the hotter weather. And that's a beautiful date to look forward to" (para. 21). Trump's optimism continued, and on February 26, 2020, Trump stated, "When you have 15 people, and the 15 within a couple of days is going to be down to close to zero, that's a pretty good job we've done," and on the next day he restated, "It's going to disappear. One day—it's like a miracle—it will disappear" (para. 22).

On March 3, 2020, Trump continued to repel the threat of coronavirus, as he stated, "It's got the world aflutter, but it'll work out," and further, Trump complained Democrats who expected him to take more actions "were perpetuating a hoax" (para. 23). On March 9, in response to this pandemic situation with 546 COVID-19 cases and twenty-two deaths in the U.S. Trump asserted there was "no reason to take drastic steps" by tweeting "Nothing is shut down, life & the economy go on" (para. 24). It is clear, according to Trump, the stability and prosperity of the economy were more important than public health. Trump withheld taking any action that would damage the operations and profits of industries. In early April 2020, Trump reiterated his priority on the economy, over public health, by stating, "Four weeks ago, we had the greatest economy in the history of the world. The greatest in the world—greatest in the history of the world" (para. 10). Trump's economy narrative explained all of his action, or lack of action, in the pandemic.

Matt Pottinger, the deputy national security adviser, concurred with the presence of Trump's economy narrative, by stating, "The Treasury and Office of Management and Budget, they were all frightened of doing anything that would disrupt the economy and so on" (*PBS*, 2020, para. 15). Trump's economy narrative prevented him from issuing a lockdown when it was necessary to do so. Fauci who was later interviewed indicated that earlier efforts to stop the spread of COVID-19 could obviously have saved lives, but the health officials had faced much pushback from the Trump administration to shut things down due to the concern of the economic impacts (Cole, 2020). When the nation went into lockdown in March, Trump continued to play down the virus. Trump wanted to reopen as soon as Easter, April 12, 2020, and "pushed states to lift restrictions early and pressured schools, churches and businesses to go back to normal, all in the hope of saving his campaign" (Karni & Haberman, 2020, para. 8).

Trump's refusal of mask-wearing was an indicator of his denial of the seriousness of the pandemic. Activities in the White House exhibited the Trump administration's continuous denial of the pandemic, projecting that it was business as usual. It was reported that "the tight quarters of the West Wing were packed and busy. Almost no one wore masks. The rare officials who did, like Matthew Pottinger, the deputy national security adviser, were ridiculed by colleagues as alarmists" (Karni & Haberman, 2020, paras. 2). Trump would order the staff who wore masks in meetings to "get that thing off" (para. 3). However, the White House's long denial of the coronavirus and the long dismissal of masks came to a sudden halt, when Trump and Melania Trump, then the first lady, and some White House staff tested positive for the virus. The Trumps' positive tests were believed to be a byproduct "of the recklessness and top-down culture of fear that Mr. Trump created at the White House and throughout his administration. If you wanted to make the boss happy, they said, you left the mask at home" (para. 7). However, after the Trumps' positive tests, mask-wearing remained optional in the White House.

Free-Rein Leadership

A leadership style is a patterned social act where an authority constructs his relationships with subordinates in an organization. The patterned social act of the authority reflects his/her understanding of his identity, the identities of the subordinates, the tasks at hand, and the goals of the organization. It is further noted that a leadership style reflects an authority's philosophy, personality, experience, and value system (Beck & Yeager, 2001; iEduNote, 2021).

What Trump chose to adopt in his response to the coronavirus pandemic was a free-rein leadership. In free-rein leadership, the person in authority gives up their power to lead and gives a high degree of freedom to the subordinates in their operations. That is, the person in authority transfers the entrusted responsibility to lead the organization to the subordinates, by giving the subordinates maximum independence in completing their assignments. Under free-rein leadership, the subordinates are given the opportunities to develop their skills, and the freedom to express their wishes, as they enjoy a high degree of autonomy and independence in their operations (Beck & Yeager, 2001; iEduNote, 2021). However, free-rein independence could easily generate fragmentations in the organization, lacking organizational cohesiveness and unity. The lack of organizational cohesion could create conflicts and chaos could occur, resulting in the loss of social objectives of the organization, and the disintegration of the organization. Without a centralized leader, the organization would operate without a clear direction, and appear to be out of control. The results could not only be inefficiency but more seriously, chaos (Beck & Yeager, 2001; iEduNote, 2021).

Despite health experts urging the White House to adopt a national strategy, a uniform approach to contain the pandemic, Trump was never clear or consistent about what the federal responsibility was, and what his responsibility was as the president of the United States. There was a lack of a unified national strategy to combat the coronavirus from the start in Trump's administration. Matt Pottinger stated, "The other thing is—really, you really have to lay at the feet of the president, there is no national plan, even to this day" (*PBS*, 2020, para. 22). Many argued for a national strategy, as the virus does not respect state borders. It was noted that techniques such as testing strategies and contact tracing, employed nationally by leaders of countries such as Germany, Italy, Greece, Vietnam, Singapore, New Zealand, and China, are standard responses in combating a pandemic; however, they were not adopted by the Trump administration. Andy Slavitt, a former federal health care official, indicated,

> They [techniques mentioned above] were not secret, . . . not mysterious. And these [countries mentioned above] were not all wealthy countries. They just

> took accountability for getting it done. But we did not do that here. There was zero chance here that we would ever have been in a situation where we would be dealing with "embers." (Shear et al., 2020, para. 99)

In March 2020, Mr. Trump informed the governors about his free-rein leadership in managing the pandemic. Lawrence Wright, a staff writer for *The New Yorker* magazine, and fellow at the Center for Law and Security at the New York University School of Law, in an interview on *PBS NewsHour*, pointed out,

> On March 11 [2020], I think it was, the president in a conversation with the 50 U.S. governors, and he said, we will be standing behind you. But then he explained what that meant. If you want to get PPE [personal protective equipment], that sort of thing, do it yourself.
>
> And, suddenly, the governors realized it wasn't a national pandemic. There were 50 epidemics. And they were totally unprepared for this. (*PBS*, 2020, paras. 23–24)

Many questioned Trump's decision to give key decisions to the states and to expect the states to take on the fight against the coronavirus by themselves, and ultimately to bring the country back to business.

In early April 2020, Trump reiterated his sideline role in the relationship of managing the pandemic between the federal government and the states as, "We're a backup. We're not an ordering clerk. We're a backup" (Woodward & Yen, 2020, para. 29). In his statement, Trump indicated that the primary responsibility for emergency supplies belonged to the states. Frances Phillips, the deputy health secretary in Maryland, stated, "It was clear that we [the state officials] were on our own and we need to develop our own strategy, which is very unlike the kind of federal response in the past public health emergencies" (Shear et al., 2020, para. 90).

However, without any coordinating efforts, states fought for medical supplies among themselves, as well as with the federal government. When the states sought support from the Strategic National Stockpile in the Health and Human Services Department—the nation's repository of medicines and other medical supplies, the federal government refused to help. Jared Kushner, the son-in-law of Trump and a senior adviser to Trump, said that "the federal stockpile is 'supposed to be our [the federal government's] stockpile.' . . . 'It's not supposed to be states' stockpiles that they then use'" (Woodward & Yen, 2020, para. 34). There is clearly a lack of solidarity, the sense of working together when facing a common threat in the country, among the states, and between the states and the federal government.

There were many incidences where Trump abdicated responsibility as the commander in chief, facing a public health emergency, even though at times he reminded others about his absolute authority as a wartime president. In April 2020, Trump stated that his role in the pandemic was similar to a "wartime president" and it would be his call about whether to reopen the country. Trump asserted, "When somebody is the president of the United States, the authority is total and that's the way it's got to be" (Shear et al., 2020, para. 52). However, a few days later, when Trump presented the guidelines to start reopening the country, the guidelines had nothing but broad, voluntary standards for states to decide how fast to come out of the lockdown, which, in political terms, meant that "[the] responsibility for dealing with the pandemic was shifting from Mr. Trump to the states" (para. 55). Indeed, Trump told the governors, "You're going to call your own shots" (para. 56). By delegating responsibilities of reopening to state governors, Trump abdicated his responsibility as the head of state in dealing with a public health emergency. Further, "during the middle weeks of April, the president's decision to largely walk away from an active leadership role—and give many states permission to believe the worst of the crisis was behind them—came abruptly into public view" (para. 51).

Many believed that Trump's free-rein leadership exhibited an intent to evade the blame when things went wrong. Although Trump has called himself "in a sense, a wartime president," and "[maximized] every opportunity to take credit for silver linings in the crisis," Trump "[did] not want to be blamed for things that go wrong" (Woodward & Yen, 2020, para. 31). Shear and associates summarized Trump's leadership dealing with the pandemic as follows:

> . . . their ultimate goal was to shift responsibility for leading the fight against the pandemic from the White House to the states. They referred to this as "state authority handoff," and it was at the heart of what would become at once a catastrophic policy blunder and an attempt to escape blame for a crisis that had engulfed the country—perhaps one of the greatest failures of presidential leadership in generations. (Shear et al., 2020, para. 3)

Discordance on the State Level

Trump pressured governors to reopen, after the lockdown had been implemented, to adhere to his economy narrative. Some governors adhered to Trump's economy narrative, pursuing economic interests, sidelining health experts, and ignoring warnings from their own advisers. Governors who adopted Trump's economy narrative often rushed to reopen and usually faced two consequences—the surge of coronavirus cases, and the discordance with the state's constituents.

Governors who adhered to Trump's economy narrative and showed inaction in the response to the coronavirus usually had the worst outbreaks. As a matter of fact, "Coronavirus cases are rising in almost every U.S. state. But the surge is worst now in places where leaders neglected to keep up forceful virus containment efforts or failed to implement basic measures like mask mandates in the first place . . . " (Leatherby & Harris, 2020, para. 1). Outbreaks were smaller in states which employed strong efforts to contain the virus in the summer and fall of 2020. In addition, it was reported that " . . . it was clear that states that rushed to reopen before meeting the criteria in the guidelines—like Arizona, Texas, and Alabama—would have among the worst surges in new cases" (Shear et al., 2020, para. 81).

In addition, governors who adhered to Trump's economy narrative often rushed to reopen schools with in-person instruction. Governors who did so faced much criticism from lawmakers and teachers. Iowa Governor Kim Reynolds is a prime example. In July 2020, when the state reported a daily record of 879 new positive Covid-19 cases, Reynolds declared that Iowa schools must prioritize in-person instruction, by conducting at least half of their instruction in-person when school reopened. Reynolds announced that "she would override local school districts and require students to spend at least half of their schooling in classrooms despite the threat to teachers, students and their families from the surge in coronavirus in the state" (Pitt, 2020, para. 1). Reynolds's announcement immediately invalidated plans which had been implemented by some school districts to limit in-person classes to one day a week, having online learning on other days. Lawmakers and teachers' union leaders criticized Reynolds's decision, stating the governor was "short-sighted for unnecessarily exposing students and school employees to a health risk . . . [and] of ignoring science and common sense" (para. 2).

The above discussion serves to illuminate Trump's economy narrative and illustrate the actions, stories, which were adopted by the Trump administration to support Trump's economy narrative. Trump's economy narrative prefigured the conflicts with Fauci, how the administration interfered with the work of the CDC, the inaction and denial adopted by Trump's free-rein leadership style, and the discordance on the state level. Although the stories might be various, the narrative was consistent throughout Trump's responses to the pandemic, the wellbeing of the economy, the trump card of Trump's re-election campaign.

BIDEN'S PUBLIC HEALTH NARRATIVE

Biden's persistent concern in regard to the pandemic was to combat COVID-19 and save lives, as illustrated in *Path Out of the Pandemic, President Biden's Covid-19 Action Plan*, a document published by the White House (https://www.whitehouse.gov/covidplan/). To do so, Biden's administration adopted a national strategy and scientific approach, absent in the previous Trump administration. The following discussion illustrates actions employed by the Biden administration, stories, to serve the persistent value in human lives in the U.S., the narrative.

Action and National Strategy

After his swearing in to office on January 20, 2021, Biden took swift actions in combating the coronavirus, reversing the actions and inactions taken by Trump. It was reported that "President Joe Biden has signed a flurry of executive orders, actions, and memorandums aimed at rapidly addressing the coronavirus pandemic and dismantling many of President Donald Trump's policies" (Sullivan, Hickey, & O'Key, 2021, para. 1). Biden had taken thirty executive orders in just three days after his swearing in to the office, more than any U.S. president in recent history. The thirty executive orders included ten executive orders that aimed at addressing the COVID-19 pandemic. The ten executive actions included imposing a mask mandate on federal property, increasing testing, organizing COVID-19 data, ramping up vaccination supplies, and requiring international travelers to provide proof of a negative COVID-19 test prior to traveling to the U.S. Biden also presented the country with the *National Strategy for the COVID-19 Response and Pandemic Preparedness*, a 200-page document aimed at combating the pandemic. Overall, "the orders signal Mr. Biden's earliest priorities in mounting a more centralized federal response to the spread of the coronavirus. Some of them mirror actions taken during the Trump administration, while most look to alter course" (Weiland, 2021b, para. 2).

A notable executive order signed by Biden, on January 21, 2021, was an executive action to require passengers to wear face coverings during interstate travel. This is a national mandate that airlines and their employees had been seeking since the beginning of the pandemic. As a contrast,

> . . . the Trump administration had refused to enact such a mask mandate, as Trump himself and many in his administration often made a point of going mask-less. The former president hosted huge rallies with like-minded supporters, often mocking Biden and others who wore masks, in spite of overwhelming evidence that properly worn face coverings significantly reduce the risk of coronavirus transmission. (Schaper, 2021, para. 4)

Without such a national mandate, some passengers had refused to follow the airlines' own mask rules. However, now under Biden's administration, it is "No Mask, No Fly."

Another notable executive order signed by Biden to reverse Trump's action was an executive action to reinstate the COVID-19 travel restrictions on non-U.S. citizens who had been in Brazil, Ireland, and the United Kingdom, and much of Europe. In addition, Biden also extended the restrictions to travelers who had recently visited South Africa. This order " . . . came just one week after President Donald Trump signed an executive order in his final days in office lifting the restrictions on travelers from these countries effective January 26 [2021]" (Saenz & LeBlanc, 2021, para. 3).

Under Trump's administration, many critics were infuriated by the inaction of Trump that had left so many needed actions undone. Vaccination was one of the major concerns, as in the Trump administration, "[in] the absence of a coordinated federal campaign, the job has fallen to overstretched, under-resourced state and local governments, with predictably wan results" (Klein, 2021, para. 4). Those critics felt relieved when the Biden administration swiftly implemented many needed actions that should have been done. Klein (2021) wrote,

> The good news is that the incoming Biden administration sees the situation clearly. "This will be one of the most challenging operational efforts ever undertaken by our country," Biden said on Friday. "You have my word that we will manage the hell out of this operation." (para. 5)

Biden's administration utilized all the available federal resources to implement combating the COVID-19 pandemic on the national level. For example,

> Biden's team members intend to use the Federal Emergency Management Agency to set up thousands of vaccination sites in gyms, sports stadiums, and community centers, and to deploy mobile vaccination options to reach those who can't travel or who live in remote places. They want to mobilize the National Guard to staff the effort and ensure that strapped states don't have to bear the cost. They want to expand who can deliver the vaccine and call up retired medical personnel to aid the campaign. They want to launch a massive public education blitz, aimed at communities skeptical of the vaccine. (para. 7)

The result was a coordinated campaign with a clear objective to save lives.

Let the Science Speak

In Biden's administration, Fauci was brought back into public view and resumed his leadership in combating the COVID-19 pandemic. After Biden was elected, in December 2020, it was announced that Fauci would serve as the Chief Medical Advisor to the President in Biden's administration. In January 2021, when the White House COVID-19 Response Team was established to replace Trump's White House Coronavirus Task Force, Fauci became a lead member of the team. On January 21, 2021, "Dr. Fauci, the nation's foremost infectious disease specialist, was back, this time with no one telling him what to say" (Shear, 2021, para. 2).

In January 2021, when Fauci was asked about the differences between working for Trump then and working for Biden now, "Dr. Fauci described the 'liberating feeling' of once again being able to 'get up here and talk about what you know—what the evidence, what the science is—and know that's it, let the science speak'" (McNeil, 2020, para. 3). Biden's appointment of Fauci to serve key roles in his administration demonstrates his belief in science and the opinions of health experts which were not valued in the previous Trump administration in combating the COVID-19 pandemic in the U.S.

Autocratic Leadership

Crisis communication calls for a leader who can act timely with clear, straightforward, and practical measures (Fearn-Banks, 2016; Coombs, 2019). To respond to the crisis of the COVID-19 pandemic, Biden did just that as he signed many executive orders to combat the pandemic in a timely fashion. By doing so, Biden adopted autocratic leadership. Using autocratic leadership, an authority leads an organization with absolute power and relates to the subordinates in extreme asymmetry. The authority dominates the decision-making and takes no account of other people's wishes or opinions. The advantage of autocratic leadership is the speed at which decisions can be made where the authority does not need to seek input from others. The fast decision-making relies on consideration of the authority and his/her core group of advisors to reach the best decision—the outcome of considering the information available at the time, the situation at hand, and the social objectives to be achieved in the organization. The decision made is mainly to achieve social objectives without compromises, pleasing, or meeting the wishes of the subordinates (Beck & Yeager, 2001; iEduNote, 2021).

Autocratic decision-making, although fast and efficient, could damage the morale of the organization as subordinates believe their needs or wishes are not accounted for. Resentment, complaints, objection, grievance, and non-compliance could occur (Beck & Yeager, 2001; iEduNote, 2021). In response to Biden's executive orders, for instance, mask mandates and vaccine mandates, complaints and objections arose (Stanley-Becker, 2021; Yan, 2021; Turner, 2021).

CONCLUSION

In responding to the coronavirus, leaders around the world adopted various strategies based on the priorities set for their countries. In the U.S. in 2020, Trump set his priority on the stability of the economy with the concern of his re-election, while his successor in 2021, Biden, set his priority on the well-being of public health. With Trump's economy narrative, there were more than four hundred thousand COVID-19 related deaths by the time Trump left office in January 2021, the highest COVID-19 death toll in the world.

Adhering to a public health narrative, Biden swiftly signed executive orders after his swearing in to the office, to implement mandates to correct the inaction of Trump's administration. Biden's action is in agreement with the discussion of leadership in crisis communication where a leader needs to act fast with decisive measures. Supporters applauded Biden's efforts in combating the pandemic and saving lives. However, due to it being an autocratic leadership, opposition arose. Objections to mask mandates and vaccination mandates were frequently reported.

REFERENCES

Abutaleb, Y., Dawsey, J., & McGinley, L. (2020, July 11). Fauci is sidelined by the White House as he steps up blunt talk on the pandemic. *The Washington Post*. Retrieved from https://www.washingtonpost.com/politics/2020/07/11/fauci-trump-coronavirus/

Beck, J., & Yeager, N. (2001). *The leader's window: Mastering the four styles of leadership to build high-performing teams* (2nd Ed.). Mountain View, CA: Nicholas Brealey America.

Behrmann, S., & Santucci, J. (2020, October 28). Here's a timeline of President Donald Trump's and Dr. Anthony Fauci's relationship. *USA Today*. Retrieved from https://www.usatoday.com/story/news/politics/2020/10/28/president-donald-trump-anthony-fauci-timeline-relationship-coronavirus-pandemic/3718797001/

CBS News. (2020, February 16). Transcript: Dr. Anthony Fauci on "Face the Nation." *CBS News*. Retrieved from https://www.cbsnews.com/news/transcript-dr-anthony-fauci-on-face-the-nation-february-16-2020/

Centers for Disease Control and Prevention (CDC). (2020, July 8). CRAFT Schools briefing packet. *The New York Times*. Retrieved from https://int.nyt.com/data/documenthelper/7072-school-reopening-packet/b70172f2cc13c9cf0e6a/optimized/full.pdf#page=1

Cohen, J. (2020, March 22). "I'm going to keep pushing." Anthony Fauci tries to make the White House listen to facts of the pandemic. *Science.org*. Retrieved from https://www.science.org/content/article/i-m-going-keep-pushing-anthony-fauci-tries-make-white-house-listen-facts-pandemic

Cole, D. (2020, April 12). Fauci admits earlier Covid-19 mitigation efforts would have saved more American lives. *CNN.* Retrieved from https://www.cnn.com/2020/04/12/politics/anthony-fauci-pushback-coronavirus-measures-cnntv/index.html

Coombs, W. (2019). *Ongoing crisis communication: Planning, managing, and responding*. Thousand Oaks, CA: Sage.

Couch, C. (1987). *Researching social processes in the laboratory*. Bingley, UK: Emerald Publishing.

Crowley, M., Thomas, K., & Haberman, M. (2020, April 5). Ignoring expert opinion, Trump again promotes use of hydroxychloroquine. *The New York Times.* Retrieved from https://www.nytimes.com/2020/04/05/us/politics/trump-hydroxychloroquine-coronavirus.html

Emma, C., & Cook, N. (2020, May 1). Fauci blocked from testifying about coronavirus response before House panel. *Politico.com.* Retrieved from https://www.politico.com/news/2020/05/01/fauci-house-panel-coronavirus-229699

Fearn-Banks, K. (2016). *Crisis communications*. New York, NY: Routledge.

iEduNote. (2021). 4 leadership styles based on authority. *iEduNote.* Retrieved from https://www.iedunote.com/leadership-styles-based-authority

Kaplan, S. (2020, October 9). White House blocked C.D.C. from requiring masks on public transportation. *The New York Times.* Retrieved from https://www.nytimes.com/2020/10/09/health/coronavirus-covid-masks-cdc.html

Karni, A., & Haberman, M. (2020, October 6). A White House long in denial confronts reality. *The New York Times.* Retrieved from https://www.nytimes.com/2020/10/03/us/politics/white-house-coronavirus.html?action=click&module=Spotlight&pgtype=Homepage

Khanna, K., & Backus, F. (2020, May 14). Trump's marks for handling COVID-19 outbreak decline—CBS News poll. *CBS News.* Retrieved from https://www.cbsnews.com/news/coronavirus-donald-trump-marks-handling-covid-outbreak-decline-cbs-news-poll-today-2020-05-14/

Klein, E. (2021, January 18). Biden's Covid-19 plan is maddeningly obvious. *The New York Times.* Retrieved from https://www.nytimes.com/2021/01/18/opinion/biden-covid-19-plan.html?action=click&module=RelatedLinks&pgtype=Article

Leatherby, L, & Harris, R. (2020, November 18). States that imposed few restrictions now have the worst outbreaks. *The New York Times.* Retrieved from https://www.nytimes.com/interactive/2020/11/18/us/covid-state-restrictions.html

Lipton, E., Sanger, D., Haberman, M., Shear, M., Mazzetti, M., & Barnes, J. (2020, July 20). He could have seen what was coming: Behind Trump's failure on the virus. *The New York Times.* Retrieved from https://www.nytimes.com/2020/04/11/us/politics/coronavirus-trump-response.html?action=click&module=RelatedLinks&pgtype=Article

Maines, D. (2001). *The faultline of consciousness: A view of interactionism in sociology*. Milton Park, UK: Routledge.

McNeil, D. (2020, January 24). Fauci on what working for Trump was really like. *The New York Times.* Retrieved from https://www.nytimes.com/2021/01/24/health/fauci-trump-covid.html

New York Times. (2020, July 24). 73,400 New Coronavirus Cases in U.S., Nearing Single-Day Record. *The New York Times.* Retrieved from https://www.nytimes.com/2020/07/24/world/coronavirus-covid-19.html?action=click&module=Top%20Stories&pgtype=Homepage#link-6ec043c9

Orr, G., & Levine, J. (2020, April 13). Trump's #FireFauci retweet spurs a cycle of outrage and a White House denial. *Politico.* Retrieved from https://www.politico.com/news/2020/04/13/trump-fauci-fire-tweet-coronavirus-183907

PBS NewsHour. (2020, December 28). Three tragic mistakes that made the 2020 pandemic worse [Video Transcript: Amna Nawaz interviews Lawrence Wright]. *PBS.* Retrieved from https://www.pbs.org/newshour/show/three-tragic-mistakes-that-made-the-2020-pandemic-worse

Page, S. (2020, May 12). The president vs. the doctor: Messages and tone conflict in a long-distance COVID-19 debate. *USA Today.* Retrieved from https://www.usatoday.com/story/news/politics/2020/ 2020/05/12/trump-vs-fauci-messages-conflict-coronavirus-readiness-reopen/3116579001/

Pitt, D. (2020, July 17). Iowa governor overrides schools, requires in-person classes. *AP News.* Retrieved from https://apnews.com/article/ecc4a3f87122f943f03fe07e37b2bf1b

Saenz, A., & LeBlanc, P. (2021, January 25). Biden reinstates Covid-19-related travel restrictions lifted by Trump. *CNN.* Retrieved from https://www.cnn.com/2021/01/24/politics/biden-coronavirus-travel-trump/index.html?utm_term=link&utm_source=fbCNNi&utm_medium=social&utm_content=2021-01-24T21%3A26%3A21&fbclid=IwAR30DTqnKYbWjLyW00TfsKfD1wPk80BsJ7qUpxecDhk1_eHhjD-kHHDSdvI

Schaper, D. (2021, January 21). No mask, no fly: Biden signs order requiring face coverings on planes. *NPR.* Retrieved from https://www.npr.org/2021/01/21/959398694/no-mask-no-fly-biden-signs-order-requiring-face-coverings-on-planes?utm_term=nprnews&utm_campaign=npr&utm_medium=social&utm_source=facebook.com&fbclid=IwAR3d11R3--cOalbUZsY2GvbyKqwNHkNhBkPGvK09cj2H7mYYxT9oUxYBLag

Shear, M. (2021, January 21). Banished by Trump but brought back by Biden, Fauci aims to "let the science speak." *The New York Times.* Retrieved from https://www.nytimes.com/2021/01/21/us/politics/fauci-trump-biden-coronavirus.html?action=click&module=Top%20Stories&pgtype=Homepage

Shear, M., Weiland, N., Lipton, E., Haberman, M., & Sanger, D. (2020, September 15). Inside Trump's failure: The rush to abandon leadership role on the virus. *The New York Times.* Retrieved from https://www.nytimes.com/2020/07/18/us/politics/trump-coronavirus-response-failure-leadership.html

Stanley-Becker, I. (2021, May 26). Resistance to vaccine mandates is building. A powerful network is helping. *The Washington Post.* Retrieved from https://www.washingtonpost.com/health/2021/05/26/vaccine-mandate-litigation-siri-glimstad-ican/?utm_campaign=wp_post_most&utm_medium=email&utm_source=newsletter&wpisrc=nl_most&carta-url=https%3A%2F%2Fs2.washingtonpost.com%2Fcar-ln-tr%2F32c4cc4%2F60ae72fc9d2fdae30261199b%2F602459d99bbc0f73f66796d4%2F9%2F70%2F60ae72fc9d2fdae30261199b

Stolberg, S. (2020, September 9). Trump administration strips C.D.C. of control of coronavirus data. *The New York Times.* Retrieved from https://www.nytimes.com/2020/07/14/us/politics/trump-cdc-coronavirus.html?campaign_id=56&emc=edit_cn_20200722&instance_id=20514&nl=on-politics-with-lisa-lerer&regi_id=83016841&segment_id=34037&te=1&user_id=0a276555af0d1325ed49414d9eb27387

Subramanian, C., Behrmann, S., & Jackson, D. (2020, February 11). Trump says Coronavirus will be gone by April when the weather gets warmer, doesn't offer scientific explanation. *USA Today.* Retrieved from https://www.usatoday.com/story/news/politics/elections/2020/02/10/trump-rallies-new-hampshire-eve-democratic-primary/4716223002/

Sullivan, K., Hickey, C., & O'Key, S. (2021, January 24). Here are the 30 executive orders and actions Biden signed in his first three days. *CNN.* Retrieved from https://www.cnn.com/2021/01/22/politics/joe-biden-executive-orders-first-week/index.html?utm_source=fbCNN&utm_medium=social&utm_term=link&utm_content=2021-01-22T16%3A45%3A08&fbclid=IwAR17G5XrVD4hZf50p8eICivHhocqHcca76KLXR4S5knxDGN0UHl84iRehxM

Turner, C. (2021, May 21). Schools are dropping mask requirements, but a new CDC study suggests they shouldn't. *NPR.* Retrieved from https://www.npr.org/2021/05/21/999106426/schools-are-dropping-mask-requirements-but-new-cdc-study-suggests-they-shouldnt?utm_medium=social&utm_source=facebook.com&utm_term=nprnews&utm_campaign=npr&fbclid=IwAR2kFGQgVdq-OvKV6djVHR7fESnYbP_2-pAE85EWWoeV_ra7lM_N3CZw15k

Weiland, N. (2021a, January 15). "Like a Hand Grasping": Trump appointees describe the crushing of the C.D.C. *The New York Times.* Retrieved from https://www.nytimes.com/2020/12/16/us/politics/cdc-trump.html

Weiland, N. (2021b, January 21). Here's what's in Biden's executive orders aimed at curbing the pandemic. *The New York Times.* Retrieved from https://www.nytimes.com/2021/01/21/us/politics/biden-executive-orders-coronavirus.html?action=click&module=Top%20Stories&pgtype=Homepage

Woodward, C., & Yen, H. (2020, April 4). AP FACT CHECK: Trump, "wartime" pandemic leader or "backup"? *PBS.* Retrieved from https://www.pbs.org/newshour/politics/ap-fact-check-trump-wartime-pandemic-leader-or-backup

Woolery, C. (2020, July 12). Twitter post [@chuckwoolery]. *Twitter.* Retrieved from https://twitter.com/chuckwoolery/status/1282499347117215745

Wu, N. (2020, July 10). Dr. Anthony Fauci says he hasn't briefed Trump in at least two months, despite pandemic resurgence. *USA Today.* Retrieved from https://www.usatoday.com/story/news/politics/2020/07/10/fauci-says-he-hasnt-briefed-trump-two-months-covid-response/5412475002/

Yan, H. (2021, May 20). The Texas governor is banning public schools from requiring masks. Here's what parents think. *CNN.* Retrieved from https://www.cnn.com/2021/05/20/us/texas-face-masks-public-schools/index.html?utm

_term=link&utm_content=2021-05-21T04%3A01%3A19&utm_source=fbCNN&utm_medium=social&fbclid=IwAR2siK_tTu9_VYHSSGSWzegICzgKn68faV_oqoaSboO8GgMcfXIHcQFoYmI

Young, M. (2020, April 11). Twitter post [@MarkYoungTruth]. *Twitter.* Retrieved from https://twitter.com/MarkYoungTruth/status/1248987423574577152

Chapter Two

Mandates vs. No Mandates

Communitarianism and Libertarianism in the Pandemic

Melissa L. Beall and Shing-Ling S. Chen

Researchers in crisis communication have indicated that in a crisis situation, an authority must act timely with clear, straightforward, and practical measures (Fearn-Banks, 2016; Coombs, 2019). To accomplish this goal, an authority usually takes on the autocratic leadership role. With autocratic leadership, an authority leads an organization with absolute power and relates to the subordinates asymmetrically. The authority dominates the decision-making, relying on his/her own observations and the input of his/her advisers.

The advantage of autocratic leadership is having the speed needed to address a crisis and to achieve the social objectives of the group. The decisions made by an autocratic leader are not meant to please other people's wishes, as the decisions are not to be compromised. Due to such a non-compromising stance of the decisions made, oppositions and complaints may arise (Beck & Yeager, 2001; iEduNote, 2021).

This is certainly the case in 2020 and 2021 in the United States during the COVID-19 pandemic. In March and April 2020, when governors issued mandatory stay-at-home orders to combat the spread of the virus, protests and complaints arose. Leading the opposition was then President Donald Trump. Trump was impatient with the lockdown orders which shut down much of the country, as he stated in a daily briefing on the COVID-19 outbreak, "We have to open our country again. We don't want to be doing this for months, and months and months" (Robb, 2020, para. 2).

In addition, there were protests staged outside of governors' mansions and state capitals across the country, in Oklahoma, Texas, Virginia, Michigan, Ohio, Kentucky, Minnesota, North Carolina, and Utah, as people were frustrated with life under lockdown (*PBS*, 2020a; Andone, 2020). Protesters, suspicious about efforts to shut down daily life to slow the spread of the virus, believed that stay-at-home orders were government overreach. Trump supported the protestors and believed some governors had gone too far on lockdown measures, despite the fact that in April 2020, the coronavirus death toll had topped forty thousand in the U.S. (Givetash, 2020).

Lockdown orders were temporary; however, some mandates are long-lasting, such as mask mandates and vaccine mandates. This chapter examines mask mandates and vaccine mandates, along with the opposition to these mandates. Such an examination sheds light on the persistent themes surrounding the mandates and their oppositions. The themes revealed allow readers to form assessments about mandates in a pandemic.

DISCORDANCE ABOUT MASK WEARING

The coronavirus is transmitted via the droplets from an infected person's cough, sneeze, or breath. Hence, mask-wearing is an effective way to slow the spread of the virus. It was reported, "Studies have shown that masks significantly decrease the chances of transmitting coronavirus, and some types of masks can help prevent their wearers from catching the virus" (Picheta, 2021, para. 4). However, in early April 2020, when the Centers for Disease Control and Prevention (CDC) urged all Americans to wear a mask when they left their home, Trump immediately undercut the message by saying, "I'm choosing not to do it" (*New York Times*, 2020, para. 2). In addition, in late April 2020, Vice President Mike Pence refused to wear a mask during his visit to the Mayo Clinic (Timm & Gregorian, 2020). Many believed that Pence's refusal to wear a mask was dangerous as an asymptomatic virus carrier could easily transmit the virus by simply having a conversation. More importantly, many believed that both Trump and Pence weakened the federal guidelines of mask-wearing by refusing to wear face coverings. In May 2020, when Trump toured the Ford car company plant in Ypsilanti, Michigan, he defied the requests from company executives to wear a face mask. To the incident, a state attorney general called Trump a "petulant child" (Walters, 2020, para. 1).

Not only did individual political leaders choose to be defiant of the CDC's mask recommendations, but people also chose to do so in large groups as well. In June 2020, at a Trump campaign rally at a church in Phoenix, few people wore masks, despite the rally being held in a coronavirus hot spot, and the church was filled to capacity with no social distancing inside (*PBS*, 2020b). In January 2021, in Des Moines, Iowa, an anti-mask protest was held at the Iowa Capitol during the first legislative session. Protestors chanted "Freedom," and held signs that stated, "Compliance is Not the Cure," "Mask Mandates Violate Bodily Autonomy," "Unmask Iowa," and "Mandates Belong in Socialist Countries" (KWWL, 2021, para. 2 & picture).

In May 2021, Iowa, Texas, and Florida forbid COVID-19 mask mandates in schools, although the CDC continued to advise face coverings in schools, medical settings, and public transit. Iowa Governor Kim Reynolds stated, "The state of Iowa is putting parents back in control of their child's education and taking greater steps to protect the rights of all Iowans to make their own healthcare decisions" (*PBS*, 2021, para. 3).

Public health officials who followed the CDC mask guidelines to implement mask mandates were reported to face violent threats on a regular basis. In June 2020, one Facebook post stated that Los Angeles County's public health director, Dr. Barbara Ferrer, should be shot (Mossburg, Waldrop, & Thomas, 2020). Also in June 2020, Nicole Quick, the former Chief Health Officer of Orange County, California, had required all residents to wear a face-covering outside their homes when it wasn't possible to keep at least six feet of distance from another person (Andrew, 2020). However, Quick quickly resigned after receiving threats of violence from the residents. Subsequently, the stricter mask mandate of requiring face covering was then changed to strongly recommending. In December 2020, Joyce Warshaw, the former Mayor of Dodge City, Kansas, after supporting a mask mandate, received so many threatening phone calls and emails from Dodge City citizens that she resigned for the concern of her own safety (Gerken & Alonso, 2020).

In June 2020, it was reported that at least twenty-four public health officials had either resigned, retired, or been fired from their positions during the COVID-19 pandemic (Mossburg, Waldrop, & Thomas, 2020). Lori Freeman, CEO of the National Association of City and County Health Officials, commented,

> What has typically been just pure public health advice coming from a trusted source in the community, the local health department, is being politicized and made to seem like the public health advice is something that is restricting people's rights, their freedoms to move about. (Mossburg, Waldrop, & Thomas, 2020, para. 8)

In November 2021, feuds over mask mandates occurred between the federal government and the state governments as well. In President Joe Biden's administration, masks were required on federal property and encouraged in schools. But Biden's order faced obstacles in several states. Florida was an example: "Most recently, Biden's Department of Education has become embroiled in a battle with Florida's Education Department after it decided to reduce funding for certain school districts for requiring people wear masks" (Picheta, 2021, para. 18).

As more businesses and states instituted mask mandates, tensions were mounting for people who saw the rules as infringements (Mervosh, Fernandez, & Robertson, 2020). Notable cases were aggressive fights that broke out on airplanes between defiant passengers who refused to wear masks and flight attendants who tried to implement airlines' mask requirements. As of this week [the week of November 28, 2021], the Federal Aviation Administration, which is responsible for enforcing the mandate on commercial flights, had reported more than 5,400 cases of unruly passenger behavior, the vast majority of which were mask-related. The agency has proposed more than $1 million in fines in connection with the incidents (Aratani, 2020, para. 4).

Defiance to mask-wearing was evident in the U.S. from individuals to groups, politicians and citizens alike. The concern for public health stipulates some to put on their masks, while the insistence on personal freedom is a major reason for not wearing a mask in public.

LEGAL BATTLES OF VACCINE MANDATES

Biden's administration issued several vaccine mandates to curb the spread of the coronavirus. However, these mandates often ran into resistance. There are two most notable mandates and their significant resistances: one issued by the Department of Labor's Occupational Safety and Health Administration (OSHA), and the other issued by the Centers for Medicare & Medicaid Services (CMS) at the Department of Health and Human Services.

OSHA Mandates for Workers

In July 2021, OSHA announced the requirement for employers with one hundred or more employees to ensure each of their workers is fully vaccinated or tests for COVID-19 on at least a weekly basis. In addition, in September 2021, Biden signed an executive order stating most federal employees must be fully vaccinated against COVID-19 and requiring large employers to have their workers inoculated or tested weekly.

In October 2021, ten states (Missouri, Nebraska, Alaska, Arkansas, Iowa, Montana, New Hampshire, North Dakota, Wyoming, and Texas) filed a joint lawsuit to challenge the Biden administration's vaccine mandate for federal contractors, a vaccine mandate that encompassed one-fifth of U.S. workers (Kornfield, Paúl, Jeong, Suliman, & Sun, 2021). Attorneys general in these states argued that the mandate infringes on states' powers and hence, is unconstitutional.

In November 2021, U.S. District Court Judge R. Stan Baker of the Southern District of Georgia stated in an order that halted the Biden administration's mandate for federal contractor employees to be vaccinated (Mulvaney, 2021). It was reported,

> The court found that the states could likely prove that Congress didn't clearly authorize the President to issue the mandate and that it "goes far beyond addressing administrative and management issues in order to promote efficiency and economy in procurement and contracting." (Mulvaney, 2021, para. 6)

However, in December 2021, the Biden administration won a battle in the appeals court. The Biden administration's mandate that requires workers at companies with one hundred or more employees to be vaccinated or undergo weekly testing, which had been blocked in November 2021, was reported to be back on (Hsu, 2021). It was reported that the Sixth Circuit Court of Appeals lifted a stay on the rule. In the lawsuits, states, businesses, religious groups, and some individuals charged the Biden administration with overreach and called the mandate an "onerous mandate" that could not be done. A three-judge panel of the Sixth Circuit believed the costs of delaying implementation of the rule to be comparatively high. Circuit Judge Jane B. Stranch, stated in the ruling,

> Fundamentally, the [rule] is an important step in curtailing the transmission of a deadly virus that has killed over 800,000 people in the United States, brought our healthcare system to its knees, forced businesses to shut down for months on end, and cost hundreds of thousands of workers their jobs. . . . The harm to the government and the public interest outweighs any irreparable injury to the individual petitioners who may be subject to a vaccination policy. (Hsu, 2021, paras. 5–6)

Iowa Governor Kim Reynolds believed that the Sixth Circuit Court made a "poor decision" allowing Biden's employer vaccination mandate to take effect, and she vowed to continue to fight against Biden's vaccine mandate for larger private employers with more than one hundred workers, affecting some eighty-four million workers in the U.S. Reynolds said, "The state has immediately asked the Supreme Court to stop this mandate, . . . I will not stop fighting for Iowans and their personal freedoms and individual liberties" (Associated Press & KWWL, 2021, para. 6). The case is now heading to the Supreme Court. At the time of this writing, the Supreme Court has begun the hearing of the arguments against the Biden administration's vaccine mandate.

CMS Mandate for Health Care Workers

In addition, CMS at the Department of Health and Human Services announced the requirement that health care workers at facilities participating in Medicare and Medicaid have to be fully vaccinated. The rule applies to more than seventeen million workers at approximately seventy-six thousand health care facilities, including hospitals and long-term care facilities.

Ten states (Iowa, Alaska, Arkansas, Kansas, Missouri, Nebraska, New Hampshire, North Dakota, South Dakota, and Wyoming) also filed lawsuits against Biden's third mandate, requiring vaccines for health care workers at facilities that get federal Medicare or Medicaid funds. In November 2021, a federal judge blocked Biden's administration from enforcing the mandate in these ten states. A federal judge in Missouri stated that the Centers for Medicare and Medicaid had no clear authority from Congress to enact the vaccine mandate for health care providers participating in the two government health care programs for the elderly, disabled, and poor (Associated Press, 2021). Iowa Governor Reynolds applauded the court's decision and stated that Iowa is fighting back against the Biden administration's attack on individual liberties. Reynolds said,

> I believe the vaccine is the best defense against COVID-19, but I also firmly believe in Iowans' right to make health care decisions based on what's best for themselves and their families, and I remain committed to protecting those freedoms. (Associated Press, 2021, para. 4)

The vaccine mandate for certain health care workers was blocked in half of the states in the country by lower courts (Sneed, 2021). The vaccine mandate is now being reviewed by the Supreme Court.

COMMUNITARIANISM AND LIBERTARIANISM

The conflicting court rulings on Biden's mandates suggest that the mandates are more than a legal issue. Mask wearing and vaccination are not merely legal issues but involve ethical concerns. The fact that the courts could not have consistent rulings, is because the courts could not rule on issues of ethics.

A consistent theme found in the arguments of anti-mask protests and anti-vaccine protestors is the protection of personal liberties. Personal liberties are certainly an important consideration when it comes to health care issues, health care issues of non-contagious diseases. For non-contagious diseases, the choice of health care is personal. However, for contagious diseases, the choice of health care is not merely personal, but social. Social wellbeing has implications on personal wellbeing, and vice versa. For contagious diseases, hence, when considering health care issues, the concern for the social, that is, the community, should supersede personal concern.

In the studies of ethics that examine the dichotomy between the community and the personal/individual, the discussion of Communitarian Ethics, as extrapolated by Clifford Christians and associates (Christians, Ferre, & Fackler, 1993), provides a guiding light. Clifford and associates emphasized the importance of the consideration of the community when one makes a decision about his/her conduct. With Communitarian Ethics, Clifford and associates believe that the community is prior to individuals and that human experiences are constructed with others within a community. According to Communitarian Ethics, human activity needs to be rooted in the community, with the concerns of others. The concerns for the community are the cornerstone of Communitarian Ethics.

Libertarianism, on the other hand, with the concern of solely oneself without the concern of the community, exhibits limitations. An individual's act, not rooted in the community, may have disastrous outcomes harming oneself and the community as well. Communitarianism is different from totalitarianism, however, where the individual's needs and concerns are not taken into consideration. Communitarianism has the components of both the community and the individuals—the individuals' needs and concerns. By pursuing common wellbeing, communitarianism also provides for the individuals and protects the individuals.

Hence, according to Communitarian Ethics, mask-wearing and vaccination take on the significance of the social meaning of pursuing communal wellbeing. They are acts of social responsibility in pursuing communal health. Without communal health, there is no personal health. With Communitarian Ethics, herd immunity, resistance to the spread of an infectious disease within a population as a result of previous vaccination, could then be achieved. By pursuing communal health, there is the protection of personal health. COVID-19 is, after all, a public health issue, not a personal health issue.

CONCLUSION

This chapter sheds light on insufficiency in the discussion of leadership in crisis communication. Crisis communication calls for a leader who acts in a timely and decisive manner. However, to meet this requirement, a leader often adopts an autocratic style of leadership which then produces opposition and resistance as seen in the previous discussions of anti-mask protests and anti-vaccine protests. The authors would like to suggest the extension of the leadership discussion in crisis communication to include the construction of a solidary relationship, as extrapolated by Carl Couch (1988). The solidary relationship created could ease the opposition and resistance in a group, and also expedite the implementation of the needed actions administered by the leader.

According to Couch, the first step of constructing a solidary relationship is to rehash the robust solidary pasts. In this case, Biden could situate the current battle with COVID-19 in the context of previous battles with contagious diseases in the U.S. such as the Spanish flu in 1918, or polio in the 1950s. By emphasizing how by working together, citizens in the U.S. triumphed in the end, after battling serious contagious illnesses.

In addition, Couch also noted that a social objective needs to be articulated in a group in order to achieve a solidary relationship. Biden, in this case, could explain to the American people the need to achieve herd immunity in order to stop the spread of COVID-19 and save lives. Couch argued that people in a solidary group do not need to agree on all the issues, but at least on one issue, the social objective, an issue with a shared interest. Hence, there may be Republicans, Democrats, Asian Americans, or African Americans in the U.S. who have their own sets of agenda to pursue; however, to stop the COVID-19 pandemic and save lives, the social objective has to be the only issue that they all agree on. Public campaigns can be used to highlight this one common goal in this diverse country.

Couch also noted the importance to treat one another with egalitarianism and altruism in a solidary group. Biden could initiate a campaign to stipulate a sense of comradery among citizens in the U.S. to promote egalitarianism and altruism in the battle against COVID-19. Brotherhood and sisterhood, as well as the intentional act to care for others, could easily be exhibited by simply wearing a mask and getting vaccinated. By introducing the construction of a solidary relationship, the discussion of leadership in crisis communication could be enhanced by removing the opposition and resistance which often comes with autocratic leadership.

REFERENCES

Andone, D. (2020, April 17). Protests are popping up across the US over stay-at-home restrictions. *CNN*. Retrieved from https://www.cnn.com/2020/04/16/us/protests-coronavirus-stay-home-orders/index.html?utm_content=2020-04-17T06%3A00%3A27&utm_source=fbCNN&utm_term=link&utm_medium=social&fbclid=IwAR2ngvIvx3HAFcrQL294c458SY8OSmuVBoV8r0cMHjJmEZL0ANo89-syYU8

Andrew, S. (2020, June 12). A California county no longer requires masks after former health officer resigns over backlash. *CNN*. Retrieved from https://www.cnn.com/2020/06/12/health/california-lifts-mask-requirement-trnd/index.html?utm_content=2020-06-12T18%3A30%3A19&utm_term=link&utm_source=fbCNN&utm_medium=social&fbclid=IwAR2U7fJvfhDGZSNKh0AIrWD-yIMdLq4muzLuyrJdE3zYNZCXNIlHLQnEkWY&fbclid=IwAR00_Y7wWzoOibDvcL6ABYUXYkowVQ3mN5BQ2kHEn1ERt1t7R56D-8XEdlA

Aratani, L. (2021, December 2). Federal mask mandate for transportation extended through March 18. *The Washington Post*. Retrieved from https://www.washingtonpost.com/transportation/2021/12/02/federal-mask-mandate-airplanes-extended/

Associated Press. (2021, November 29). Biden vaccine rule for health workers blocked in Iowa, 9 other states. *The Gazette*. Retrieved from http://www.thegazette.com/health-care-medicine/biden-vaccine-rule-for-health-workers-blocked-in-iowa-9-other-states/

Associated Press and KWWL. (2021, December 17). Gov Reynolds: Court made "poor decision" allowing Biden employer vaccine mandate to take effect. *KWWL*. Retrieved from https://www.kwwl.com/news/politics/gov-reynolds-court-made-poor-decision-allowing-biden-employer-vaccine-mandate-to-take-effect/article_99770645-c4e7-52b5-831b-f7cd7938f23d.html?fbclid=IwAR0FW6-4QYdeX23I4vq2VUWkhR6x2ECuYql7lFA3RMqchAmEoHUUJ0QwAGw

Beck, J., & Yeager N. (2001). *The leader's window: Mastering the four styles of leadership to build high-performing teams*, 2nd Edition. Mountain View, CA: Nicholas Brealey America.

Christians, C., Ferre, J., & Fackler, P. (1993). *Good news: Social ethics and the press*. New York: Oxford University Press.

Coombs, W. (2019). *Ongoing crisis communication: Planning, managing, and responding*. Thousand Oaks, CA: Sage.

Couch, C. (1988). *Social processes and relationships*. Dix Hills, NY: General Hall.

Fearn-Banks, K. (2016). *Crisis communications*. New York, NY: Routledge.

Gerken, M., & Alonso M. (December 20, 2020). A mayor received so many threats after supporting a mask mandate that she resigned. *CNN*. Retrieved from https://www.cnn.com/2020/12/16/us/mayor-resigns-over-masks-trnd/index.html

Givetash, L. (2020, April 11). Coronavirus: Trump says some governors "have gone too far" on lockdown measures. *NBC News*. Retrieved from https://www.nbcnews.com/news/world/coronavirus-trump-says-some-governors-have-gone-too-far-lockdown-n1187596?fbclid=IwAR1_vdt239rmfJK2Ym4l7tC_dxRoD5wujaNQDDpZW3Jbh30tINztINzASUc

Hsu, A. (2021, December 18). Biden's vaccine-or-test rule for 84 million workers is back after court lifts stay. *NPR*. Retrieved from https://www.npr.org/2021/12/17/1065401498/bidens-osha-vaccine-mandate-test-million-workers?utm_term=nprnews&utm_campaign=npr&utm_medium=social&utm_source=facebook.com&fbclid=IwAR1wjevTr1dk6HkNwFz9BtTJA5K5Dmh-p6vOXM0nchpS7cFyhLwWVpB4GSQ

iEduNote. (2021). 4 Leadership Styles Based on Authority. *iEduNote*. Retrieved from https://www.iedunote.com/leadership-styles-based-authority

Kornfield, M., Paúl, M., Jeong, A., Suliman, A., & Sun, L. (2021, October 29). More than 10 GOP states sue Biden administration over vaccine mandates. *The Washington Post*. Retrieved from https://www.washingtonpost.com/nation/2021/10/29/covid-delta-variant-live-updates/

KWWL. (2021, January 11). Anti-mask protest held at Iowa Capitol during first legislative session. *KWWL*. Retrieved from https://kwwl.com/2021/01/11/anti-mask-protest-held-at-iowa-capitol-during-first-legislative-session/?fbclid=IwAR3OdoiUVVXdxG7sSxwQzjKoLpPXEYJtvnkPNNbjli1kK323WXWXyBenoOr

Mervosh, S., Fernandez, M., & Robertson, C. (2020, July 16). Mask rules expand across U.S. as clashes over the mandates intensify. *The New York Times*. Retrieved from https://www.nytimes.com/2020/07/16/us/coronavirus-masks.html?action=click&module=Well&pgtype=Homepage&section=US%20News

Mossburg, C., Waldrop T., & Thomas N. (2020, June 23). Some public health officials are resigning amid threats during the Covid-19 pandemic. *CNN*. Retrieved from https://www.cnn.com/2020/06/22/us/health-officials-threats-coronavirus/index.html?utm_term=link&utm_content=2020-06-23T04%3A00%3A15&utm_medium=social&utm_source=fbCNN&fbclid=IwAR2L5fWLw2EbNDkw0kkFSZdTADzIgG8qv95AzInS7syrlitZUjpdTwM4S_8

Mulvaney, E. (2021, December 7). Biden vaccine mandate for federal contractors is blocked nationwide. *Bloomberg*. Retrieved from https://www.bloomberg.com/news/articles/2021-12-07/biden-vaccine-mandate-for-federal-contractors-blocked-nationwide

New York Times. (2020, April 3). Coronavirus live updates: C.D.C. recommends wearing masks in public; Trump says, "I'm Choosing Not to Do It." *The New York Times*. Retrieved from https://www.nytimes.com/2020/04/03/world/coronavirus-news-updates.html?action=click&module=Spotlight&pgtype=Homepage

PBS. (2020a, April 17). Pro-Trump protesters push back on stay-at-home orders. *PBS*. Retrieved from https://www.pbs.org/newshour/nation/pro-trump-protesters-push-back-on-stay-at-home-orders?fbclid=IwAR0k2OssNzBlNBl14fiv2qnjm4j5FvmLLORHXKvtpMwnuG3pHl5evWdwR2A

PBS. (2020b, June 23). Trump's Phoenix speech brings thousands together indoors—in a virus hot spot. *PBS*. Retrieved from https://www.pbs.org/newshour/show/trumps-phoenix-speech-brings-thousands-together-indoors-in-a-virus-hot-spot?fbclid=IwAR3VQSGqGb7ZFYySkwZEERmpLM4nC7ikOTGins3BsO--zCGYcj0yxwyfGaw

Picheta, R. (2021, November 2). Why the world is still arguing over face masks, 20 months into the pandemic. *CNN*. Retrieved from https://www.cnn.com/2021/11/02/health/face-mask-debate-covid-19-pandemic-cmd-intl/index.html?utm_medium=social&utm_content=2021-11-02T09%3A30%3A06&utm_term=link&utm_source=fbCNNi&fbclid=IwAR3sDq40h2xZFq4hKOAz2gL1jKUCM_F2WL1xdGjRR3_BWOgCkSYK2rkLjUk

Reuters. (2021, May 20). Iowa joins U.S. states forbidding COVID-19 mask mandates in schools. *Reuters*. Retrieved from https://www.reuters.com/business

/healthcare-pharmaceuticals/iowa-joins-us-states-forbidding-covid-19-mask-mandates-schools-2021-05-20/

Robb, G. (2020, April 5). "We have to open our country again," says Trump, even as he warns of "a lot of death" in coming weeks. *Market Watch*. Retrieved from https://www.marketwatch.com/story/we-have-to-open-our-country-again-says-trump-showing-impatience-with-stay-home-orders-2020-04-04

Sneed, T. (2021, December 18). Appeals court lets Biden administration enforce vaccine rules for large employers. *CNN*. Retrieved from https://www.cnn.com/2021/12/17/politics/appeals-court-vaccine-mandate-osha-large-employers-federal-contractors/index.html

Timm, J., & Gregorian, D. (2020, April 29). "Dangerous & disrespectful": Doctors tear into Pence's mask-less hospital visit. *NBC News*. Retrieved from https://www.nbcnews.com/politics/white-house/dangerous-disrespectful-doctors-tear-pence-s-mask-less-hospital-visit-n1195611

Walters, J. (2020, May 22). Donald Trump goes without mask at Michigan Ford plant despite company request. *The Guardian*. Retrieved from https://www.theguardian.com/us-news/2020/may/21/trump-ford-factory-mask-michigan

Chapter Three

Religious Freedom vs. Public Health

Discordant Legal Narratives in the Pandemic

Juliet Dee

- March 2020: Members of the Skagit Valley Chorale attend a two-hour choir practice at Mount Vernon Presbyterian Church in Mount Vernon, Washington. Of the sixty-one singers who attend, fifty-three later test positive for the coronavirus; two of them die (Baker, 2020).
- March 2020: Several members of the Faith Presbyterian Church in Sacramento, California, attend church services and later test positive for the coronavirus; two of them die (Hooks & Tieu, 2020).
- March 2020: Among ninety-four people who attend a church in rural Arkansas, thirty-five test positive for the coronavirus; three of them die (James et al., 2020).
- March 2020: Among two hundred bishops and pastors who attend the Eastern Kansas Minister's Conference at Miracle Temple Church of God in Christ in Kansas City, Kansas, fifty-one test positive for the coronavirus; seven of them die (KCTV-5, 2020).
- June 2020: Seventeen-year-old Carsyn Davis attends a church youth group gathering with more than one hundred teenagers at the First Assembly of God in Fort Myers, Florida. Few if any teens are wearing face masks. Carsyn Davis contracts the coronavirus and dies (Czachor, 2020).
- October 2020: Approximately one thousand people attend services at the United House of Prayer for All People in Charlotte, North Carolina.

> They do not wear facemasks and there is no social distancing. A few weeks later, 213 people test positive for the coronavirus and twelve people die (Mazziotta, 2020).

With the outbreak of the coronavirus pandemic in March 2020, public health officials across the United States scrambled to put social-distancing requirements in place, and state governors issued lockdown orders to "flatten the curve" and try to prevent the virus from spreading so rapidly. These lockdown orders instigated discordant responses from religious leaders. The issue here, framed as "Religious Freedom vs. Public Health: Discordant Legal Narratives in the Pandemic," led to hundreds of religious leaders filing lawsuits against their state governments, arguing that they had the right to conduct religious services in person. At first, most religious leaders deferred to lockdown orders and streamed their services via Zoom. When leaders of some churches and synagogues defied lockdown orders, they argued that the lockdowns violated the Establishment Clause of the First Amendment. In other words, they argued that orders restricting church or synagogue attendance to ten, twenty-five, or fifty people violated the free exercise of their religion. Courts have struggled to balance the rights of free exercise of religion and freedom of assembly against the rights of governors to issue regulations to protect public health. The "free exercise of religion" clause is part of the First Amendment, which holds that "Congress shall make no law respecting an establishment of religion, or prohibiting the free exercise thereof" (Free Exercise Clause, 1791).

The need for courts to find the appropriate balance between conflicting constitutional rights raises the larger question of how "paternalistic" Americans want their government to be. For example, as a society, we accept laws requiring us to wear seatbelts, laws requiring motorcyclists to have helmets, and laws requiring people on boats to have life jackets. However, many Americans have balked at requirements to wear facemasks and refrain from gathering in groups of ten or more, suggesting that they did *not* want federal or state governments to try to protect them.

This chapter will analyze the legal arguments in cases in which judges have tried to balance the conflicting claims of free exercise of religion, freedom of assembly, and the right of local, state, and federal officials to enforce regulations to protect public health. Judges have applied the *ad hoc balancing theory* of First Amendment law in deciding these cases, meaning that they make their decisions on a case-by-case basis, depending on the unique facts of each case. The problem with the *ad hoc balancing theory* is that it is difficult for attorneys, plaintiffs, and defendants to predict how judges will rule in any given case. We saw the U.S. Supreme Court uphold California's lockdown restrictions against gathering in churches and synagogues, but then we saw it strike down New York's restrictions against gathering in churches and synagogues six months later; to say that court decisions have been discordant is an understatement.

DISCORD AMONG FEDERAL VERSUS STATE AND CITY GOVERNMENTS

During Spring 2020, there were often conflicting messages from federal, state, and local governments. Former President Donald Trump at first declared the coronavirus to be "a hoax" and later suggested that people could kill the virus with hydroxychloroquine or perhaps by injecting bleach or ultraviolet light into their bloodstreams (Clark, 2020). Despite Dr. Anthony Fauci's pleas for Americans to wear facemasks and shelter at home, Trump called Dr. Fauci "an alarmist" and refused to have the federal government mandate the wearing of facemasks. During an interview with Fox News correspondent Chris Wallace, Trump said of the coronavirus: "It's going to disappear. I'll be right, because I've been right [about the coronavirus] probably more than anybody else" (Rogers, 2020, para. 15).

On May 22, 2020, Trump declared:

> Houses of worship, churches, synagogues and mosques are essential places that provide essential services. Some governors have deemed liquor stores and abortion clinics as essential, but have left out churches and other houses of worship. It's not right, so I'm correcting this injustice and calling houses of worship essential. . . . If [the governors] don't do it, I will override the governors. In America, we need more prayer, not less. (Forgey, Roubein, & Ward, 2020, paras. 2–3, 13)

Trump faced immediate pushback from state and local officials, however. Rhode Island Governor Gina Raimondo and Chicago Mayor Lori Lightfoot questioned whether Trump had the power to override local authorities; Lightfoot said: "By no means can the President order any locality, any state to do something that he doesn't have the power to do. And he can't do that here" (Forgey, Roubein, & Ward, 2020, para. 8).

Complicating matters further, nearly thirty years ago Congress passed the *Religious Freedom Restoration Act of 1993 (RFRA)* (1993), which includes the section *"Free Exercise of Religion Protected"* (1993). In 2017 then–Attorney General Jeff Sessions issued the Memorandum *"Federal Law Protections for Religious Liberty,"* which emphasized that the Department of Justice would enforce the RFRA (Attorney General, 2017). Of course this preceded the onslaught of the coronavirus. The RFRA holds that the federal government may not interfere with a person's free exercise of religion unless there is (1) a compelling government interest (keeping people from dying from the coronavirus) and (2) "the least restrictive means of furthering that [compelling] interest" (Free Exercise of Religion Protected, 1993, § 2000bb–1). Although *everyone* would no doubt agree that preventing individuals from dying of the coronavirus *is* a compelling government interest, the question of whether or not limiting houses of worship to ten people or fewer comprised the "least restrictive means" has become an issue resulting in litigation across the country. The *Religious Freedom Restoration Act* applies not only to the federal government, and twenty-one state legislatures have passed similar statutes.

Relying on the "free exercise of religion" clause of the First Amendment and the *Religious Freedom Restoration Act*, Donald Trump asked Attorney General William Barr to intervene on behalf of churches that filed lawsuits against governors' lockdown restrictions. For example, in April 2020, members of Greenville, Mississippi's Temple Baptist Church attended a drive-in service at which they stayed in their parked cars with windows rolled up to hear their pastor Arthur Scott's sermon. However, the City of Greenville had prohibited drive-in church services, so police arrived, knocked on car windows, and wrote citations with $500 fines. Barr directed the U.S. Department of Justice to intervene; its attorneys argued that the City of Greenville's restrictions were "neither neutral nor generally applicable" (Temple Baptist Church v. City of Greenville, 2020a, p. 8). In other words, the Justice Department argued that the City of Greenville was discriminating against houses of worship as compared with "essential" businesses such as restaurants; for example, Attorney General Barr argued that it made no sense for the City of Greenville to permit its citizens "to sit in a car at a drive-in restaurant with their windows rolled *down*, but not at a drive-in church service with their windows rolled *up*" (Temple Baptist Church v. City of Greenville, 2020a, p. 9). In August 2020, the City of Greenville lifted its restrictions and permitted drive-in church services; thus, a federal district court judge dismissed the church's case against the City of Greenville (Temple Baptist Church v. City of Greenville, 2020b).

Just as William Barr had intervened on behalf of the Temple Baptist Church (Temple Baptist Church v. City of Greenville, 2020a), he intervened on behalf of the Lighthouse Fellowship Church on Chincoteague Island in Virginia in May 2020. Police cited the church during a Palm Sunday celebration in April 2020 after sixteen people attended an in-person service because Virginia's limit for in-person religious services was ten people. The police issued a criminal summons to Pastor Kevin Wilson, charging him with violating Virginia Governor Ralph Northam's executive order, a misdemeanor that could carry a penalty of one year in jail and a $2,500 fine. Lighthouse Fellowship Church identified itself as a church "providing hope for people who are hurt, broken, and discarded" (Velazquez, 2020, para. 4). Its congregants included recovering drug addicts and former prostitutes. The church filed suit against Virginia Governor Ralph Northam, but in May 2020, a federal district court judge upheld Governor Northam's executive order; in his conclusion he explained: "These restraints [on in-person gatherings] have been imposed for the common good to slow the spread of the novel coronavirus and to save the lives of countless people" (Lighthouse Fellowship Church v. Ralph Northam, 2020a, p. 442). The U.S. Department of Justice then filed a Statement in Support of Plaintiff (Lighthouse); then–Vice President Mike Pence also spoke publicly in Pastor Kevin Wilson's defense. The federal district court again upheld Governor Northam's executive order (Lighthouse Fellowship Church v. Ralph Northam, 2020b), at which point the church appealed to the U.S. Court of Appeals for the Fourth Circuit. After Governor Northam issued a new executive order that exempted houses of worship from the ten-person limit for indoor services, however, the Fourth Circuit dismissed the church's case as moot (Lighthouse Fellowship Church v. Ralph Northam, 2020c).

The *Temple Baptist Church* and *Lighthouse Fellowship Church* cases in which the U.S. Department of Justice intervened highlight the disagreement among state governors and the federal government regarding whether or not religious services were "essential." In spring 2020, states were literally "all over the map," meaning that some governors declined to order lockdowns, or if they *did* ask their citizens to stay at home, their lockdown orders did not apply to houses of worship. For example, Texas Governor Greg Abbott designated houses of worship as "essential," meaning that they could remain open without restrictions (Abbott, 2020). New Mexico's Governor Michelle Grisham allowed people to gather in houses of worship even after she had locked down movie theatres and concert halls. Ohio's General Assembly passed a law that prohibited public officials such as the governor from closing houses of worship (General Assembly of the State of Ohio, 2019–2020). After Kansas Governor Laura Kelly issued an executive order limiting religious gatherings to no more than ten people in April 2020, the Legislative Coordinating Council of the Kansas state legislature revoked Governor Kelly's executive order, at which point she asked the state Supreme Court to intervene. She explained that at first, she had exempted houses of worship from her lockdown restrictions, but when seven bishops and pastors died of the coronavirus after attending a conference of the Church of God in Christ in Kansas City, Governor Kelly amended her executive order to include houses of worship. The Kansas Supreme Court held that the Legislative Coordinating

Council of the state legislature did not have the authority to revoke Governor Kelly's lockdown restrictions; thus it upheld her executive order that limited in-person religious services to ten people or fewer (Kelly v. Legislative Coordinating Council, 2020).

California had no limits on the number of people who could gather for religious services outdoors, but after conducting a fifty-state survey of restrictions on indoor worship, the Becket Fund for Religious Liberty noted that California was "the only state to ban indoor worship altogether" (Becket Fund, 2021, pp. iii, 18).

There were fifteen states, specifically, Arizona, Arkansas, Colorado, Florida, Georgia, Michigan, North Dakota, Ohio, Pennsylvania, South Carolina, South Dakota, Tennessee, Texas, Utah, and West Virginia, which held that religious gatherings were exempt from any attendance limitations. In contrast, the other thirty-five states imposed restrictions ranging from banning all in-person religious gatherings to setting limits of ten, twenty-five, or fifty members of a congregation who could be present in person (Szymanski, 2021).

In addition to urging state governors to designate houses of worship as "essential," Donald Trump also sought out states and churches that might provide him with a sympathetic audience. In May 2020, Trump held a jamboree in which three thousand Republican college students gathered at the Dream City Church in Phoenix, Arizona; they sat next to each other and only a few wore facemasks. The young adults may have felt safe because the church's pastors had explained that the company Clean Air EXP had installed a new "magic air system" that would "neutralize 99.9% of the coronavirus within 10 minutes" (Medina & Chang, 2020, para. 1). Dream City Church officials and the event organizer, Turning Point Action, may have had doubts about the "magic air," however. They required everyone who registered for the event to sign a waiver that said, "By attending this convention, you . . . voluntarily assume all risks related to exposure to COVID-19 and agree not to hold Turning Point Action . . . liable for any illness or injury" (Medina & Chang, 2020, para. 25). Arizona's Attorney General Mark Brnovich later sent a cease-and-desist letter to Clean Air EXP and Dream City Church, demanding that they stop making false claims about a "magic" air purification system.

ARGUMENTS FOR ATTENDING HOUSES OF WORSHIP IN PERSON

Catholic, Protestant, and Jewish religious leaders soon filed lawsuits against their state governors, arguing that "drive-in" services, in which parishioners stayed in their cars in the parking lot, or services via Zoom were unacceptable; they argued that they had to conduct services in person. For example, Father Trevor Burfitt filed suit against California Governor Gavin Newsom after Newsom had banned houses of worship from holding indoor services, although there was no limit on the number of people who could attend outdoor religious services. Burfitt's attorneys expressed shock and dismay at being forced outdoors, and criticized the impact of Newsom's restrictions on Father Burfitt's constitutional rights, typically in the following two paragraphs:

> 219. the Catholic Mass is ordered to the temple, not the outdoors. A Catholic church is focused entirely upon the Holy Sanctuary where Christ in the Blessed Sacrament resides in the Tabernacle. Neither the Tabernacle nor the Catholic Mass belongs in a parking lot or other outdoor location, which lend themselves to the desacralization of the sacred mysteries and profanation of the Blessed Sacrament. Yet [Governor] Newsom has forced Father Burfitt and his congregations outdoors while innumerable "essential" business activities are conducted indoors under Newsom's ever-more elaborate web of permissions and prohibitions. To be forced by a mere politician to offer the sacred mystery of the Holy Sacrifice of the Mass outside of God's temple is in itself to undergo religious persecution by the State.
>
> 220. Nor is there any possibility of worshipping "remotely" by "streaming or other technologies that support physical distancing and state public health guidelines." It is a foundational Catholic tenet that one cannot receive Sacraments without being physically present for their administration, as the Sacraments themselves consist of both matter and form. Sacraments cannot confer their benefits by video link. "Virtual worship" deprives Catholics of the incalculable benefits of divine grace as conferred through the Church's bimillennial Sacramental forms, instituted by Christ Himself. (Burfitt v. Newsom, Complaint, 2020, p. 55)

Just as Father Burfitt argued in California that Catholics had to attend Mass in person, when New York limited the number of people who could attend an indoor religious service to ten, upstate New York Catholic priests Steven Soos and Nicholas Stamos filed suit against then-Governor Andrew Cuomo. Soos and Stamos argued that if Catholics do not attend Mass in person each week, they are committing a "mortal sin," meaning that they will burn in hell for eternity, but if only ten people could attend Mass, the priests would have to hold more Masses per day than was possible. They further argued that drive-in Masses were unacceptable because Catholics must kneel while receiving Holy Communion; thus Governor Cuomo's executive orders "prohibit reception of Holy Communion itself—the very essence of the Mass" (Soos v. Cuomo, 2020, p. 276).

Soos and Stamos were co-plaintiffs with Daniel Schonbrun, Elchanan Perr, and Mayer Mayerfeld, members of Orthodox Jewish synagogues in Brooklyn, New York. Schonbrun, Perr, and Mayerfeld explained to the court that "the synagogue prayers must have a minimum quorum of ten adult men called the *minyan.*" With the ten-person limit, although Schonbrun, Perr, and Mayerfeld could attend services if they were part of the quorum, their wives and children were excluded because only ten men could be in the synagogue at one time. They further argued that drive-in synagogue services were unacceptable because "the minyan must all be present in the same room, not in various motor vehicles, . . . [m]oreover, any type of operation of a vehicle is prohibited on the Sabbath" (Soos v. Cuomo, 2020, p. 277). Pastor Mark Anthony "Tony" Spell filed suit against Louisiana Governor John Bel Edwards's executive order restricting in-person church attendance to ten people or fewer (Spell v. Edwards, 2020a, 2020b). He explained his religious beliefs that "baptisms, communion, the laying on of hands, and anointing the sick with oil must be done in person in a church assembly" (Spell v. Edwards, 2020a, p. 2). As law professor Michael Conklin explains:

> Religious institutions feared that weeks and perhaps months without in-person monetary collections would be a potentially crippling, if not mortal, blow. Some religious adherents believed that they would be "divinely protected," and that the COVID-19 pandemic did not absolve their obligation to attend in-person religious services. Others pointed to the religious aspects of loving thy neighbor through protecting the health of others. (Conklin, 2020, p. 65)

DISCORD AMONG RELIGIOUS LEADERS AND POLICE

In Spring 2020 a number of pastors openly defied their governors' lockdown orders and continued to hold in-person church services with far more than ten people. For example, in March 2020 Pastor Dan Ostring of the Rivers of Living Waters church in Sacramento, California, continued to hold in-person services each week and posted videos of his services on YouTube; in one of the videos, Pastor Ostring said: "Welcome to another Sunday civil disobedience act. We were told to stay home. Do not go to church. You might get sick. I ain't never seen such fear mongering in my life" [sic] (Hooks & Tieu, 2020, para. 22). In April 2020 several police officers met Pastor Jon Duncan of the Cross Culture Christian Center in Lodi, California, to inform him that he could not hold an in-person service on Palm Sunday (Branson-Potts, 2020).

After one thousand people attended an in-person service at the Life Tabernacle Church in Baton Rouge, Louisiana in March 2020, police issued a summons to Pastor Tony Spell (mentioned above, Spell v. Edwards, 2020a,

2020b) for violating Governor John Bel Edwards's executive order limiting houses of worship to in-person services with no more than ten people. Police also arrested Pastor Spell for trying to hit a protestor with one of Spell's church buses (Mitchell, 2020). Also in March 2020, State Attorney Andrew Warren warned Pastor Rodney Howard-Browne of the River at Tampa Bay Church in Florida not to hold services with more than ten people, but Howard-Browne ignored the warnings and held services with nine hundred people, at which point police arrested him and charged him with violating public health emergency regulations. Discussing the arrest, State Attorney Warren explained:

> I'd remind the good pastor of Mark 12:31, which said there's no more important commandment than to love thy neighbor as thyself. Loving your neighbors is protecting them, not jeopardizing their health by exposing them to this deadly virus. (Marrero, 2020, para. 9)

A week after police arrested Howard-Browne, Florida Governor Ron DeSantis changed his executive order to exempt all houses of worship from the ten-person limit, and prosecutors later dropped the charges against Howard-Browne (Marrero, 2020).

Although police arrested a few pastors across the country, the preferred means of resistance to governors' lockdown restrictions was through the courts; houses of worship filed lawsuits, arguing that lockdown restrictions were infringing on their "free exercise of religion" that the First Amendment guarantees. Some of the legal challenges came from the Christian Right; social scientist Jeffrey Haynes explains:

> The Christian Right was alarmed that their religious freedoms were being curtailed—albeit temporarily—in order to fight the pandemic. Many did not accept the medical reasons behind the closures of places of religious worship; instead, some regarded the closures as sinister: an aspect of secularization whose purpose, they believed, was to undermine and eventually remove the right of religious believers to exercise their faith. . . . Others refused to believe that COVID-19 was "real," contending instead that it was a "phantom plague." (Haynes, 2021, p. 6)

Thus, with legal teams such as Liberty Counsel and the Alliance Defending Freedom, the Christian Right initiated many (but not all) of the lawsuits challenging state governors' lockdown restrictions on houses of worship.

SOUTH BAY UNITED PENTECOSTAL CHURCH SETS THE PRECEDENT

In mid-May 2020 Bishop Arthur Hodges of the South Bay United Pentecostal Church joined forces with Rabbi Mendel Polichenco of Chabad of Carmel Valley (both in the San Diego area) to file suit against California Governor Gavin Newsom. They argued that California's stay-at-home orders banning in-person religious services were a violation of the Establishment Clause of the First Amendment. Bishop Hodges explained that assembling in person was important for the several hundred people in his congregation: "For example, it's essential for people to be baptized. But you can't baptize yourself. You have to have the church, the clergy, to do that" (NBC-7, 2020, para. 12). Their attorneys requested an injunction to prevent the state of California from enforcing the lockdown against houses of worship, and their case quickly reached the U.S. Supreme Court.

In reaching their decision, the Justices of the U.S. Supreme Court accorded great weight to the legal precedent *Jacobson v. Commonwealth of Massachusetts* (1905), cited in *South Bay United Pentecostal Church v. Newsom* (2020b, pp. 1613–1614). In *Jacobson*, during an ongoing smallpox epidemic, Swedish Lutheran minister Henning Jacobson challenged a state law requiring compulsory vaccination against smallpox. Since Jacobson refused to be vaccinated, he had to pay a $5 fine. In 1905, the High Court upheld the authority of Cambridge, Massachusetts to require compulsory vaccination. The Justices explained that no constitutional right was absolute, and that individual liberty does not extend to harming others:

> Upon the principle . . . of paramount necessity, a community has the right to protect itself against an epidemic of disease which threatens the safety of its members. To safeguard that end, states may delegate their public health powers to Boards of Health. (Jacobson v. Commonwealth of Massachusetts, 1905, p. 27)

The Justices of the U.S. Supreme Court denied South Bay's application for injunctive relief, citing *Jacobson* (1905) and *Marshall v. United States* (1974):

> . . . Our Constitution principally entrusts "[t]he safety and the health of the people" to the politically accountable officials of the States to "guard and protect." *Jacobson v. Massachusetts* [citation omitted] (1905). When those officials "undertake to act in areas fraught with medical and scientific uncertainties," their latitude "must be especially broad." *Marshall v. United States* [citation omitted] (1974). (South Bay United Pentecostal Church v. Newsom, 2020b, p. 1613)

In a case similar to *Jacobson,* the U.S. Supreme Court held that "the right to practice religion freely does not include liberty to expose the community or the child to communicable disease, . . . ill health or death" (Prince v. Commonwealth of Massachusetts, 1944, para. 16).

After a federal district court upheld Governor Newsom's lockdown restrictions, Bishop Hodges and Rabbi Polichenco turned to the U.S. Court of Appeals for the Ninth Circuit. The appellate court likewise upheld California's restrictions; in their opinion, the Ninth Circuit judges commented that a court should not "convert the constitutional Bill of Rights into a suicide pact" (South Bay United Pentecostal Church v. Newsom, 2020a, p. 939).

In *South Bay,* Chief Justice John Roberts cited *Jacobson* in his concurring opinion; Justices Stephen Breyer, Ruth Bader Ginsburg, Sonia Sotomayor, and Elena Kagan agreed with Chief Justice Roberts, but Justice Brett Kavanaugh wrote a dissent that Justices Clarence Thomas, Samuel Alito, and Neil Gorsuch joined. The 5–4 majority held that judges should defer to public health officials' advice to governors during the coronavirus pandemic; thus, they upheld California's lockdown in late May 2020, ruling against Bishop Hodges's and Rabbi Polichenco's request to hold in-person services (South Bay United Pentecostal Church v. Newsom, 2020b). *South Bay* set the precedent in similar California cases; for example, when the Harvest Rock Church in Pasadena challenged Governor Newsom's ban on all indoor services in houses of worship, a federal district court again upheld California's lockdown restrictions (Harvest Rock Church v. Newsom, 2020).

Between May and November 2020, more than one hundred lower court judges relied on Chief Justice John Roberts's concurring opinion in *South Bay* and upheld lockdown restrictions in their jurisdictions (see Parmet, 2020, pp. 1042–1048, for a list of all lawsuits filed by houses of worship from March through May 2020), but other lower courts relied on Kavanaugh's dissent. As law professor Wendy Parmet (2020) explains, "the lower courts diverged over how to reconcile the deference that *Jacobson* accords to public health authorities with the protection of fundamental constitutional rights" (p. 1002). For example, when the rural church Calvary Chapel Dayton Valley filed suit against Nevada Governor Steve Sisolak, Calvary Chapel argued that Sisolak's restrictions permitting only fifty people to meet in person in a church were unfair in view of the fact that Las Vegas casinos were permitted to have 50 percent of their capacity (which could easily exceed fifty people). In a 5–4 opinion, the justices upheld Governor Sisolak's restrictions, citing *South Bay.* Justice Samuel Alito dissented:

> The Constitution guarantees the free exercise of religion. It says nothing about the freedom to play craps or blackjack, to feed tokens into a slot machine or to

engage in any other game of chance. But the Governor of Nevada apparently has different priorities. (Calvary Chapel Dayton Valley v. Sisolak, 2020, p. 1)

A SPLIT AMONG THE CIRCUITS

Like Justice Alito, not all lower court judges agreed with *South Bay* and *Calvary Chapel Dayton Valley*. In the federal court system, there are ninety-four federal district courts organized in twelve circuits. Each circuit has its own court of appeals that reviews cases decided in the federal district courts if litigants appeal from the lower court decision. Although it is rare, if a panel of judges in one circuit hands down a decision that conflicts with a decision in another circuit, this results in the dreaded "split between the circuits," and only the U.S. Supreme Court can resolve issues in which appellate courts arrive at differing conclusions. For example, the U.S. Courts of Appeal for the Fifth and Sixth Circuits ruled in favor of churches re-opening, whereas the U.S. Courts of Appeal for the Second, Seventh, and Ninth Circuits upheld governors' lockdown orders limiting in-person attendance in houses of worship.

Fifth and Sixth Circuits Strike Down Restrictions on Houses of Worship

In April 2020, police in Mississippi interrupted an Easter Sunday service and issued a citation to members of the First Pentecostal Church of Holly Springs, advising them that they could hold drive-in but not in-person church services. In response, fifty members of the church, none of them wearing face masks but dressed in their Sunday best, staged a protest in which they paraded through the aisles of a WalMart to make the point that fifty of them could be indoors in a store but not in a church. After WalMart security guards asked them to vacate the premises because they were not there to shop, they gathered outside the store where their minister praised the Lord (Watson, 2020). Pastor Jerry Waldrop then sued the City of Holly Springs, demanding the right to hold in-person services. Federal district court Judge Michael Mills asked if it was "worth risking the very lives of their fellow congregants and other members of the community? Unfortunately, [the church] and its members appear to have decided that the answer to this question is 'yes' . . . " (First Pentecostal Church of Holly Springs v. City of Holly Springs, 2020a, p. 2). Judge Mills acknowledged that Mississippi Governor Tate Reeves had designated churches as "essential," but he added:

> This court is unclear . . . and it has generally had considerable difficulty in ascertaining what is and is not permitted under Governor Reeves' executive orders, as it relates to church services. (p. 3)
>
> This court is by no means certain on this point [whether churches could have in-person services] . . . and it has contacted the Governor's legal staff to request that he submit an amicus brief setting forth his position on this issue. (p. 4)
>
> This entire lawsuit is nothing more than a deeply misguided attempt on [the church's] part to gain permission to endanger their own lives and those of their fellow community members. (p. 8)

Judge Mills expressed concern about the fact that fifty church members had staged a protest at a local WalMart:

> . . . no pretense was given that the church members were actually shopping during the visit, and they apparently were comfortable in subjecting actual shoppers with potential exposure to a deadly virus merely to make a point in this litigation. . . . This court considers the visit [to the WalMart] to have been highly reckless in light of the ongoing pandemic. (p. 9)
>
> In these times, when a pandemic stalks the world, this court realizes that decisions regarding previously mundane matters may be deadly. (p. 11)

Not satisfied with Judge Mills's hesitation, Pastor Waldrop filed an appeal with the U.S. Court of Appeals for the Fifth Circuit, which ruled in the church's favor, enjoining the City of Holly Springs from enforcing its order against in-person services. The case was in effect moot, however. A few days before the Fifth Circuit's decision, an arsonist burned the church to the ground and spray-painted graffiti in the parking lot that said: "Bet you stay home now, you hypokrits [sic]" (First Pentecostal Church of Holly Springs v. City of Holly Springs, 2020b, p. 670).

Whereas Mississippi Governor Tate had issued "Safe Worship Guidelines for In-Person Worship Services" (First Pentecostal Church of Holly Springs v. City of Holly Springs, 2020b, p. 670), in Kentucky (the Sixth Circuit's jurisdiction), Governor Andy Beshear ordered all houses of worship to close because they were not "life-sustaining." Governor Beshear ruled that law firms, laundromats, liquor stores, and gun shops *did* qualify as "life-sustaining," however (Maryville Baptist Church v. Beshear, 2020, p. 611). Ironically, houses of worship could remain open to provide soup kitchens, homeless shelters, and "social services," but could not meet in person for religious services (p. 611). In spring 2020, the Maryville Baptist Church was one of the several different churches that filed suit against Kentucky's lockdown regulations; a few of the other lawsuits were *On Fire Christian Center v. Fischer* (2020), *Roberts v. Neace* (2020), and *Tabernacle Baptist Church v. Beshear* (2020).

Of these cases, *On Fire Christian Center* is aptly named; federal district court Judge Justin Walker himself was "on fire" in writing his opinion. This case began in April 2020 when Louisville Mayor Greg Fischer notified all churches that they could hold neither in-person nor even drive-in services on Easter Sunday, even if parishioners remained in their cars. The On Fire Christian Center asked for a temporary restraining order (TRO) which would enjoin the City of Louisville from prohibiting drive-in church services on Easter Sunday, and Judge Walker immediately granted it. Judge Walker (On Fire Christian Center v. Fischer, 2020) noted On Fire's effort to maintain social distancing and indicated that "On Fire has planned a drive-in church service in accordance with the Center for Disease Control's social distancing guidelines" (p. 909), which required that "cars will park six feet apart and all congregants will remain in their cars with windows no more than half open for the entirety of the service. . . ." (p. 911). He explained his judgment on this matter:

> On Holy Thursday an American mayor criminalized the communal celebration of Easter. That sentence is one that this Court never expected to see outside the pages of a dystopian novel, or perhaps the pages of *The Onion*. But two days ago, citing the need for social distancing during the current pandemic, Louisville's Mayor Greg Fischer ordered Christians not to attend Sunday services, even if they remained in their cars to worship—and even though it's Easter. The Mayor's decision is stunning. And it is, beyond all reason, unconstitutional. (p. 905)

Following a discussion of persecuted Christians beginning with St. Paul and the Pilgrims, Judge Walker zeroed in on the question of what comprised "essential" businesses that the City of Louisville permitted to remain open:

> Those "essential" activities include driving through a liquor store's pick-up window, parking in a liquor store's parking lot, or walking into a liquor store where other customers are shopping. The Court does not mean to impugn the perfectly legal business of selling alcohol, nor the legal and widely enjoyed activity of drinking it. But if beer is "essential," so is Easter. (p. 911)

Just ten days after Judge Walker ruled in favor of the On Fire Christian Center, Mayor Greg Fischer and the church reached an out-of-court settlement in which the City of Louisville permitted drive-in church services after all.

In contrast to Judge Walker, however, federal district court Judge David Hale ruled against Kentucky's Maryville Baptist Church, which had held a drive-in service on Easter Sunday. At this drive-in service, the police walked up to each car and "issued notices to the congregants that their attendance at the drive-in service amounted to a criminal act" (Maryville

Baptist Church v. Beshear, 2020, p. 611). After Judge Hale upheld Governor Beshear's restrictions, the church filed an appeal with the U.S. Court of Appeals for the Sixth Circuit, which reversed Judge Hale's decision, ruling that Governor Beshear's order had violated the Free Exercise Clause of the First Amendment (Maryville Baptist Church v. Beshear, 2020, p. 611). In the related case of *Roberts v. Neace* (2020), Maryville Baptist Church parishioner Theodore Roberts filed suit against Boone County Attorney Robert Neace and Governor Beshear, claiming that when police had placed the "attendance-is-criminal" notices on their car, it violated their Free Exercise rights. Again, the Sixth Circuit ruled in Roberts's favor. It held that the state of Kentucky could not show preferential treatment for "life-sustaining" businesses such as grocery stores over "soul-sustaining" houses of worship. Law professor Wendy Parmet (2020) comments on the appellate court's decisions:

> [The Sixth Circuit] did not consider any public health evidence. . . . Rather than look to science, the court relied solely on its own common sense conclusion. As a result, the court failed to consider that many of the distinctions that [the state of Kentucky] drew made sense based on what was known at the time about the virus. Gatherings of many people in a building for an extended period of time are likely far more dangerous than the more transient encounters in retail establishments. Further, communal prayer and singing may add to the risk . . . [however] the Sixth Circuit felt no need to defer to [public health officials] or be informed by the science. (pp. 1028–1029)

Seventh Circuit Follows Ninth Circuit Precedent

In contrast to the Fifth and Sixth Circuits' rulings in favor of houses of worship holding in-person services, the U.S. Court of Appeals for the Seventh Circuit upheld Illinois Governor Jay Robert Pritzker's Executive Order 2020–32; this limited house of worship attendance to ten people or fewer. The Elim Romanian Pentecostal Church challenged Governor Pritzker's order, arguing that in-person fellowship was an essential element of its parishioners' faith. The federal district court held that the solution was to have multiple separate church services with ten persons or fewer, and the Seventh Circuit affirmed the lower court's decision. The Seventh Circuit also emphasized that it was following the precedent set in Chief Justice John Roberts's concurring opinion in *South Bay,* in which he held that churches and concert halls were in a category different from "essential" businesses such as grocery stores and pharmacies:

> We line up with Chief Justice Roberts. . . . As Chief Justice Roberts observed, concerts and church services differ from grocery stores and pharmacies, "in which people neither congregate in large groups nor remain in close

proximity for extended periods." (Elim Romanian Pentecostal Church v. Pritzker, 2020, p. 10)

The Seventh Circuit explained that Governor Pritzker's Executive Order 2020–32 was a "law of general application," meaning that it applied to *everyone,* and did not discriminate against any religion.

ROMAN CATHOLIC DIOCESE 0F BROOKLYN V. CUOMO REVERSES *SOUTH BAY*

The U.S. Supreme Court changed course from its *South Bay* "super-precedent" when it struck down New York's lockdown regulations for religious institutions. In October 2020, then-Governor Andrew Cuomo imposed a color-coded "Cluster Action Initiative" that imposed more stringent restrictions on "Red Zone" areas with higher coronavirus rates; in Red Zones, houses of worship were limited to in-person services of ten people or fewer. The Roman Catholic Diocese of Brooklyn had churches in Brooklyn and Queens, some of which could seat from seven hundred to one thousand people. Agudath Israel, with Orthodox Jewish synagogues in both boroughs, at least one of which could seat four hundred people, challenged the restrictions in court. The federal district court judges upheld New York State's Red Zone restrictions (Roman Catholic Diocese of Brooklyn v. Cuomo, 2020a; Agudath Israel v. Cuomo, 2020), and the U.S. Court of Appeals for the Second Circuit affirmed.

The Roman Catholic Diocese of Brooklyn and Agudath Israel both appealed to the U.S. Supreme Court in November 2020. In September 2020 Justice Ruth Bader Ginsburg had passed away, and Justice Amy Coney Barrett took her place, creating a new conservative majority (Justices Clarence Thomas, Samuel Alito, Neil Gorsuch, Brett Kavanaugh, and Amy Coney Barrett) with a liberal minority (Chief Justice John Roberts and Justices Stephen Breyer, Sonia Sotomayor, and Elena Kagan). The High Court noted that although houses of worship in Red Zones had a hard limit of ten people, "essential" secular businesses such as grocery stores had no limit on the number of people that could be indoors in Red Zones. The majority emphasized that it was addressing the question for all fifty states, not just New York: "In recent months, certain other governors have issued similar edicts [to New York's Red Zone restrictions]. At the flick of a pen, they have asserted the right to privilege restaurants, marijuana dispensaries, and casinos over churches, mosques, and temples" (Roman Catholic Diocese of Brooklyn v. Cuomo, 2020b, p. 69). The majority continued: "It is hard to believe that admitting more than ten people to a 1,000-seat church or 400-seat synagogue would create a more serious health risk than the many other activities that the State allows" (p. 67). The majority rejected the argument that religious services via Zoom were an adequate substitute: "Catholics who watch a Mass at home cannot receive communion, and there are important religious traditions in the Orthodox Jewish faith that require personal attendance" (p. 68).

The majority now rejected *South Bay,* arguing that this decision "was mistaken from the start. [The *South Bay* decision] reached back one hundred years . . . to *Jacobson v. Massachusetts,* but *Jacobson* hardly supports cutting the Constitution loose during a pandemic" (Roman Catholic Diocese of Brooklyn v. Cuomo, 2020b, p. 70). The High Court thus held that the Roman Catholic Diocese of Brooklyn and Orthodox Jewish synagogues could hold in-person services with more than ten congregants. This comprised a seismic shift in the High Court's direction; in the months following *Roman Catholic Diocese,* the majority has consistently ruled in favor of "free exercise of religion" over governors' attempts to maintain lockdowns during the coronavirus pandemic.

THE TIDE TURNS IN FAVOR OF HOUSES OF WORSHIP

A few weeks later, South Bay United Pentecostal Church, along with Harvest Rock Church in California, again challenged Governor Gavin Newsom's restrictions on holding religious services indoors in light of *Roman Catholic Diocese.* However, the federal court and the U.S. Court of Appeals for the Ninth Circuit distinguished *Roman Catholic Diocese,* and continued to uphold Governor Newsom's orders against indoor religious services. The Ninth Circuit reasoned that although California did not permit indoor services, state regulations permitted an unlimited number of people to gather for outdoor religious services (because it is always sunny in California). Both South Bay and Harvest Rock appealed to the U.S. Supreme Court, and in February 2021, the High Court ruled in the two churches' favor, ruling that Governor Newsom could not rely on California's "mild climate" to mandate outdoor services only. In other words, California had to permit indoor worship services in accordance with *Roman Catholic Diocese* (South Bay United Pentecostal Church v. Newsom, 2021 [South Bay II]; Harvest Rock Church v. Newsom, 2021 [Harvest Rock II]).

Because California prohibited indoor private gatherings and restricted outdoor gatherings to three households, Pastor Jeremy Wong and Karen Busch filed suit against Governor Newsom, demanding that they be permitted to hold Bible studies, theological discussions, and "musical prayer" at their homes. Although a federal district court and the Ninth Circuit had upheld California's restrictions, the U.S. Supreme Court reversed in April 2021, citing *Roman Catholic Diocese*; thus, Wong and Busch were allowed to hold worship services in their homes (Tandon v. Newsom, 2021).

Encouraged by *Roman Catholic Diocese,* the rural Nevada church Calvary Chapel Dayton Valley again filed a legal challenge to Nevada's lockdown, and in December 2020, the Ninth Circuit struck down the fifty-person limit on house-of-worship attendance. In June 2021 the state of Nevada agreed to pay $175,000 in attorneys' fees to the Alliance Defending Freedom, which had represented Calvary Chapel Dayton Valley in court (Sonner, 2021). At the same time, the state of California agreed to pay $1.6 million in attorneys' fees to South Bay United Pentecostal Church, $1.35 million in attorneys' fees to Harvest Rock Church (Coleman, 2021), and $550,000 in attorneys' fees to Father Trevor Burfitt of the Society of Saint Pius X (a total of $2.15 million). The state of California also agreed to a permanent injunction that prohibited Governor Newsom from imposing restrictions on houses of worship after the U.S. Supreme Court had struck down such restrictions in *Roman Catholic Diocese* (Davis, 2021).

DISCUSSION

Law professor Jeff Thaler (2021) asks: "When confronting an emergency, to what extent can the government curtail civil rights?" (p. 207). And legal scholar Josh Blackman (2021) asks: "Did the [government] have the power to restrict religious assembly, but permit other types of commercial gatherings?" (p. 760). Legal scholars Lindsay Wiley and Stephen Vladek (2020) warn that permitting state governments to institute draconian restrictions could threaten civil liberties in the future. In contrast, legal scholar Caroline Corbin (2020) argues that state governments *should* have the power to restrict indoor religious gatherings because houses of worship "where people talk, sing and socialize are high-risk and are potential super-spreader events. While that generally does not describe people at their local supermarket or even liquor store, it *does* describe religious services" (p. 26). Law professor Daniel Farber (2020) cautions that "there is no magic formula for striking the balance" between the need for deference to public health officials' guidelines during a pandemic and the courts' duty to protect constitutional rights such as the free exercise of religion (p. 863).

From March to November 2020, the U.S. Supreme Court and lower courts appeared to apply the *ad hoc balancing theory* of the First Amendment; in other words, they balanced the Establishment Clause's guarantee of free exercise of religion against the need for government officials to protect public health through social distancing. In November 2020, however, the U.S. Supreme Court in essence overturned its *South Bay* decision and adopted the *preferred position balancing theory* in *Roman Catholic Diocese.* The preferred position balancing theory rests on the assumption that First Amendment freedoms are fundamental to a democratic society and should receive greater judicial protection when certain rights come into conflict. In other words, in *Roman Catholic Diocese,* the High Court gave preference to the free exercise of religion over state governments' efforts to maintain social distancing to prevent the spread of the coronavirus. The U.S. Supreme Court majority in *Roman Catholic Diocese* also seemed troubled by the fact that state governors were allowing retail establishments such as grocery stores to remain open with more than ten shoppers at one time. In other words, the majority believed that limiting churches and synagogues to only ten people placed an unfair "burden" on the free exercise of religion.

In view of the fact that pastors, priests, and rabbis filed hundreds of lawsuits against their state governors, demanding the right to have in-person religious services, it is clear that communal, in-person worship is of huge importance to some individuals. The coronavirus lockdowns caused enormous discord among religious leaders and public health officials who were desperately trying to prevent the coronavirus from spreading. Before the Pfizer, Moderna, and Johnson & Johnson vaccines were available, if patients were dying from the coronavirus, doctors and nurses had to isolate these patients; their families could not be with them in the hospital. As of this writing, more than 985,000 Americans have died of the coronavirus since March 2020. Before the vaccines were available, if individuals attended an in-person religious service, they might have enjoyed worshipping with others, but if they caught the coronavirus while they were there, they would die alone.

REFERENCES

Abbott, G. (2020, April 27). Executive Order GA-18 relating to the expanded reopening of services as part of the safe, strategic plan to open Texas in response to the COVID-19 disaster. *The Governor of the State of Texas*. Retrieved from https://gov.texas.gov/uploads/files/press/EO-GA-18_expanded_reopening_of_services_COVID-19.pdf

Agudath Israel of America v. Andrew M. Cuomo, No. 20–3572-CV [Docket No. 20A90], U.S. Court of Appeals for the 2nd Circuit (2020). Retrieved from https://www.supremecourt.gov/search.aspx?filename=/docket/docketfiles/html/public/20a90.html

Attorney General. (2017, October 26, effective November 27). Federal Law Protections for Religious Liberty. FR Doc. 2017–23338 [Fed Reg. Vol. 82, No. 206, at 49672]. *Department of Justice*. Retrieved from https://www.govinfo.gov/content/pkg/FR-2017-10-26/pdf/2017-23269.pdf

Baker, S. (2020, May 13). An infamous Washington choir practice led to 53 COVID-19 cases and 2 deaths—and could have been down to a "super-emitter" in the choir. *Business Insider.* Retrieved from https://www.businessinsider.com/coronavirus-cdc-says-washington-choir-session-53-cases-2-deaths-2020-5

Becket Fund for Religious Liberty. (2021, January). Motion for leave to file brief *amicus curiae* in support of applicants by the Becket Fund for Religious Liberty, *South Bay United Pentecostal Church v. Newsom, Harvest Rock Church v. Newsom,* Nos. 20A136 & 20A137, U.S. Supreme Court. Retrieved from https://www.supremecourt.gov/DocketPDF/20/20A136/167600/20210129103806958_South%20Bay%20and%20Harvest%20Rock%20Amicus%20FINAL.pdf

Blackman, J. (2021, Summer). The "essential" free exercise clause. *Harvard Journal of Law & Public Policy*, *44*(3), 637–760. Retrieved from https://www.harvard-jlpp.com/wp-content/uploads/sites/21/2021/06/Blackman-The-Essential-Free-Exercise-Clause.pdf

Branson-Potts, H. (2020, April 5). Pastor who refuses to cancel Sunday services because of coronavirus greeted by police. *Los Angeles Times.* Retrieved from https://www.latimes.com/california/story/2020-04-05/pastor-who-refuses-to-cancel-sunday-services-greeted-by-police

Burfitt v. Newsom, No. BCV-20–102267 [Complaint for Declaratory and Injunctive Relief], Superior Court of the State of California, County of Kern, Metro Division (2020). Retrieved from https://www.thomasmoresociety.org/wp-content/uploads/2020/10/California-Fr.-Burfitt-Complaint.pdf

Calvary Chapel Dayton Valley v. Steve Sisolak, Docket No. 19A1070 [On Application for Injunctive Relief], U.S. Supreme Court (2020, July 24). Retrieved from https://www.supremecourt.gov/opinions/19pdf/19a1070_08l1.pdf#page=13

Clark, D. (2020, April 23). Trump suggests "injection" of disinfectant to beat coronavirus and "clean" the lungs. *NBC News.* Retrieved from https://perma.cc/R6DC-BJ4Y

Coleman, A. (2021, May 17). Harvest Rock Church wins lawsuit: Restrictions on houses of worship banned; state must reimburse church legal fees. *Pasadena Now.* Retrieved from https://www.pasadenanow.com/main/harvest-rock-church-newsom-reach-settlement/

Conklin, M. (2020). The most demanding test known to Constitutional law: Do COVID-19 bans on church services satisfy Religious Freedom Restoration Act requirements? *Washburn Law Journal*, *60*(1), 63–76. Retrieved from https://contentdm.washburnlaw.edu/digital/collection/wlj/id/7277/rec/61

Corbin, C. M. (2020). Religious liberty in a pandemic. *Duke Law Journal Online*, *70*(September), 1–28. Retrieved from https://scholarship.law.duke.edu/cgi/viewcontent.cgi?article=1080&context=dlj_online

Czachor, E. (2020, July 6). Florida teen who contracted coronavirus dies after mother took her to church party, then treated her with hydroxychloroquine. *Newsweek.* Retrieved from https://www.newsweek.com/florida-teen-dies-after-mother-took-her-church-coronavirus-party-then-treated-her-1515781

Davis, K. (2021, June 2). State to pay $2.15 million in attorney fees in COVID-19 church lawsuits: The settlement also lays out guidelines prohibiting similar worship restrictions. *The San Diego Union-Tribune.* Retrieved from https://www.sandiegouniontribune.com/news/courts/story/2021-06-02/state-covid-19-church-lawsuits

Elim Romanian Pentecostal Church v. J. B. Pritzker, Case No. 20–1811, U. S. Court of Appeals, Seventh Circuit (2020, June 16). Retrieved from http://media.ca7.uscourts.gov/cgi-bin/rssExec.pl?Submit=Display&Path=Y2020/D06-16/C:20-1811:J:Easterbrook:aut:T:fnOp:N:2531757:S:0

Farber, D. (2020). The long shadow of Jacobson v. Massachusetts: Public health, fundamental rights and the courts. *San Diego Law Review, 57*(4), 833–863. Retrieved from https://digital.sandiego.edu/sdlr/vol57/iss4/1/

First Pentecostal Church of Holly Springs v. City of Holly Springs, Mississippi, CASE NO. 3:20CV119 M-P, U.S. District Court for the Northern District of Mississippi, Oxford Division (2020a, May 14). Retrieved from https://casetext.com/case/first-pentecostal-church-of-holly-springs-v-city-of-holly-springs

First Pentecostal Church of Holly Springs v. City of Holly Springs, Mississippi, 959 F. 3d 669 [No. 20–60399], U.S. Court of Appeals, Seventh Circuit (2020b, May 22). Retrieved from https://scholar.google.com/scholar_case?case=18013740506504638025&hl=en&as_sdt=6&as_vis=1&oi=scholarr

Forgey, Q., Roubein, R., & Ward, M. (2020, May 22). Trump declares houses of worship "essential," pressuring governors to let them re-open. *Politico.* Retrieved from https://www.politico.com/news/2020/05/22/trump-churches-essential-coronavirus-274763

Free Exercise Clause. (1791). United States Constitution, Amendment I.

Free Exercise of Religion Protected. 42 U.S. Code (The Public Health and Welfare) § 2000bb-1. (1993). Retrieved from https://www.law.cornell.edu/uscode/text/42/2000bb-1

General Assembly of the State of Ohio. (2019–2020). Expand court jurisdiction to any constitutional basis. Ohio House Bill 272, 133rd Gen. Assembly, Regular Session. Retrieved from https://legiscan.com/OH/text/HB272/2019/

Harvest Rock Church, Inc., et al. v. Gavin Newsom, No. 20–55907, U. S. Court of Appeals, Ninth Circuit (2020). [Harvest Rock I]. Retrieved from https://cdn.ca9.uscourts.gov/datastore/opinions/2020/10/01/20-55907.pdf

Harvest Rock Church, Inc., et al. v. Gavin Newsom, 141 S.Ct. 1289 [No. 20–55907], U.S. Supreme Court (2021). [Harvest Rock II]. Retrieved from https://scholar.google.com/scholar_case?case=9174364450728365255&hl=en&as_sdt=6&as_vis=1&oi=scholarr

Haynes, J. (2021, January 30). Donald Trump, the Christian right and COVID-19: The politics of religious freedom. *Laws 2021, 10*(1), 6. Retrieved from https://www.mdpi.com/2075-471X/10/1/6/htm

Hooks, K., & Tieu, V. (2020, April 2). Church says Sacramento County's reporting of 71 members infected with coronavirus are "believed to be inaccurate." *ABC-10.* Retrieved from https://www.abc10.com/article/news/health/coronavirus/three-pastors-among-71-infected-at-sacramento-church/103-96db2e21-5eaf-4ebf-8643-4c4aa8c65b6e

Jacobson v. Commonwealth of Massachusetts, 197 U.S. 11 [25 S.Ct. 358; 49 L.Ed. 643], U.S. Supreme Court (1905). Retrieved from https://supreme.justia.com/cases/federal/us/197/11/

James, A., Eagle, L., Phillips, C., Hedges, D. S., Bodenhamer, C., Brown, R., Wheeler, J. G., & Kirking, H. (2020, May 22). High COVID-19 attack rate among attendees at events at a church—Arkansas, March 2020. Centers for Disease Control and Prevention. *Morbidity & Mortality Weekly Report (MMWR) 69*(20), 632–635. Retrieved from https://www.cdc.gov/mmwr/volumes/69/wr/mm6920e2.htm

KCTV-5. (2020, April 20). 7 deaths, 51 COVID-19 cases related to Kansas City, Kansas church gathering. *KCTV News*. Retrieved from https://www.kctv5.com/coronavirus/7-deaths-51-covid-19-cases-related-to-kck-church-gathering/article_7ad23784-833c-11ea-b588-d7dd9fad8338.html

Kelly v. Legislative Coordinating Council, Kansas House of Representatives & Kansas Senate, No. 122,765, Supreme Court of the State of Kansas (2020). Retrieved from https://www.kscourts.org/Cases-Opinions/Opinions/Published/Kelly-v-Legislative-Coordinating-Council

Lighthouse Fellowship Church v. Northam, 458 F. Supp. 3d 418, U.S. District Court, E.D. Virginia, Norfolk Division (2020a, May 1). Retrieved from https://scholar.google.com/scholar_case?case=4461103304725908568&hl=en&as_sdt=6&as_vis=1&oi=scholarr

Lighthouse Fellowship Church v. Northam, 462 F. Supp. 3d 635, U.S. District Court, E.D. Virginia, Norfolk Division (2020b, May 21). Retrieved from https://scholar.google.com/scholar_case?case=16877244971204854891&hl=en&as_sdt=6&as_vis=1&oi=scholarr

Lighthouse Fellowship Church v. Northam, No. 20–1515, U.S. Court of Appeals, Fourth Circuit (2020c, October 13). *2020 U.S. App. LEXIS 33377*. Retrieved from https://advance-lexis-com.udel.idm.oclc.org/document/documentlink/?pdmfid=1516831&crid=13222b13-c6a3-4d4b-a83d-fd6ee3e7702d&pddocfullpath=%2Fshared%2Fdocument%2Fcases%2Furn%3AcontentItem%3A614C-GFJ1-JX3N-B1F3-00000-00&pdcontentcomponentid=6388&pddoctitle=Lighthouse+Fellowship+Church+v.+Northam%2C+2020+U.S.+App.+LEXIS+33377+(4th+Cir.%2C+Oct.+13%2C+2020)&pdproductcontenttypeid=urn%3Apct%3A30&pdiskwicview=false&ecomp=sswvk&prid=1157b954-eb59-44f5-b7f7-fdeb06bcabe9

Marrero, T. (2020, May 15). Charges dropped against Tampa pastor who held services during stay-at-home order. *Tampa Bay Times*. Retrieved from https://www.tampabay.com/news/health/2020/05/15/charges-dropped-against-tampa-pastor-who-held-services-during-stay-at-home-order/

Marshall v. United States, 414 U.S. 417 [94 S.Ct. 700; 38 L.Ed.2d 618], U.S. Supreme Court (1974). Retrieved from https://supreme.justia.com/cases/federal/us/414/417/

Maryville Baptist Church v. Beshear, 957 F. 310 610, U.S. Court of Appeals, Sixth Circuit (2020). Retrieved from https://scholar.google.com/scholar_case?case=3713654395071230391&hl=en&as_sdt=6&as_vis=1&oi=scholarr

Mazziotta, J. (2020, November 30). COVID outbreak at North Carolina church linked to 12 deaths and more than 200 cases. *People*. Retrieved from https://people.com/health/covid-outbreak-north-carolina-church-linked-12-deaths-200-cases/

Medina, J., & Chang, K. (2020, June 24). Ahead of Trump visit, church makes unproven claim of virus-killing technology. *New York Times.* Retrieved from https://www.nytimes.com/2020/06/23/us/politics/trump-arizona-church-covid.html

Mitchell, D. J. (2020, May 15). Judge rejects Central pastor's lawsuit against governor; he is released from house arrest. *The Advocate.* Retrieved from https://www.theadvocate.com/baton_rouge/news/coronavirus/article_d9657b70-9710-11ea-bfa5-1b911fa7e233.html

NBC-7. (2020, May 14). South Bay Bishop suing county, state: "We've passed point where government can impose emergency order." *NBC-7 San Diego.* Retrieved from https://www.nbcsandiego.com/news/local/south-bay-bishop-suing-county-state-weve-passed-point-where-govt-can-impose-emergency-order/2325515/

On Fire Christian Center v. Fischer, 453 F. Supp. 3d 901, U. S. District Court, Western District of Kentucky (2020, April 11). Retrieved from https://scholar.google.com/scholar_case?case=13036323887025481426&hl=en&as_sdt=6&as_vis=1&oi=scholarr

Parmet, W. E. (2020). The COVID cases: A preliminary assessment of judicial review of public health powers during a partisan and polarized pandemic. *San Diego Law Review*, *57*(4), 999–1048. Retrieved from https://digital.sandiego.edu/cgi/viewcontent.cgi?article=3394&context=sdlr

Prince v. Commonwealth of Massachusetts, 321 U.S. 158, U.S. Supreme Court (1944). Retrieved from https://www.law.cornell.edu/supremecourt/text/321/158

Religious Freedom Restoration Act of 1993 (RFRA). Pub. L. 103–141. 42 U.S. Code 2000bb-1(a)(b). (The Public Health and Welfare) Chapter 21B (1993). Retrieved from https://www.law.cornell.edu/uscode/text/42/chapter-21B

Roberts v. Neace, 958 F. 3d 409, U.S. Court of Appeals, Sixth Circuit (2020). Retrieved from https://scholar.google.com/scholar_case?case=8449531878915252666&hl=en&as_sdt=6&as_vis=1&oi=scholarr

Rogers, K. (2020, July 19). Trump leans into false virus claims in combative Fox News interview. *New York Times.* Retrieved from https://www.nytimes.com/2020/07/19/us/politics/trump-fox-interview-coronavirus-race.html

Roman Catholic Diocese of Brooklyn v. Cuomo, No. 20-cv-4844(NGG)(CLP), U.S. District Court, E.D. New York (2020a, October 9). Retrieved from https://scholar.google.com/scholar_case?case=16666251904841887727&hl=en&as_sdt=6&as_vis=1&oi=scholarr

Roman Catholic Diocese of Brooklyn v. Cuomo, 141 S.Ct. 63, U.S. Supreme Court (2020b, November 25). Retrieved from https://scholar.google.com/scholar_case?case=14249141472030529264&hl=en&as_sdt=6&as_vis=1&oi=scholarr

Sonner, S. (2021, June 23). One Nevada church settles; other pressing COVID-19 lawsuit. *U.S. News.* Retrieved from https://www.usnews.com/news/best-states/nevada/articles/2021-06-23/one-nevada-church-settles-other-pressing-covid-19-lawsuit

Soos v. Cuomo, 470 F. Supp. 3d. 268, U.S. District Court, Northern District of New York (2020, June 26). Retrieved from https://scholar.google.com/scholar_case?case=14226261059760097765&hl=en&as_sdt=6&as_vis=1&oi=scholarr

South Bay United Pentecostal Church v. Newsom, 959 F. 3d 938, U.S. Court of Appeals, Ninth Circuit (2020a, May 22). Retrieved from https://scholar.google.com/scholar_case?case=15477914146509879049&hl=en&as_sdt=6&as_vis=1&oi=scholarr

South Bay United Pentecostal Church v. Newsom, 140 S. Ct. 1613, U.S. Supreme Court (2020b, May 29). Retrieved from https://scholar.google.com/scholar_case?case=5226635228340381841&hl=en&as_sdt=6&as_vis=1&oi=scholarr

South Bay United Pentecostal Church v. Newsom, 141 S. Ct. 716, U.S. Supreme Court (2021) [South Bay II]. Retrieved from https://scholar.google.com/scholar_case?case=14593292829267142959&hl=en&as_sdt=6&as_vis=1&oi=scholarr

Spell v. Edwards. (2020a, November 11). Emergency application for writ of injunction pending appellate and certiorari review. *Wittenbrink Law Firm*. Retrieved from https://www.supremecourt.gov/DocketPDF/20/20A91/160370/20201111173741112_Application%20and%20Appendix%20-%20Spell%20v.%20Edwards.pdf

Spell v. Edwards, No. 20A91. U.S. Supreme Court (2020b, November 18). Retrieved from https://www.supremecourt.gov/search.aspx?filename=/docket/docketfiles/html/public/20a91.html

Szymanski, J. M. (2021, April 26). Tracking faith-based legal challenges to pandemic orders: How federal courts nationwide are addressing religious liberty arguments by churches. *Church Law & Tax*. Retrieved from https://www.churchlawandtax.com/web/2020/may/tracking-pandemic-related-religious-liberty-cases.html

Tabernacle Baptist Church v. Beshear, 459 F. Supp. 3d 847, U.S. District Court, Eastern District of Kentucky, Central Division, Frankfort (2020). Retrieved from https://scholar.google.com/scholar_case?case=15496188851517795076&hl=en&as_sdt=6&as_vis=1&oi=scholarr

Tandon v. Newsom, 141 S. Ct. 1294, U.S. Supreme Court (2021). Retrieved from https://scholar.google.com/scholar_case?case=17656243762288077494&hl=en&as_sdt=6&as_vis=1&oi=scholarr

Temple Baptist Church v. City of Greenville, No. 4:20-CV-64-DMB-JMV [The United States Statement of Interest in Support of Plaintiffs]. U.S. District Court, Northern District of Mississippi (2020a, April 14). Retrieved from https://www.justice.gov/opa/press-release/file/1268651/download

Temple Baptist Church v. City of Greenville, No. 4:20-CV-64-DMB-JMV [Order Closing Case], U.S. District Court, Northern District of Mississippi, Greenville Division (2020b, August 13). Retrieved from https://scholar.google.com/scholar_case?case=5498868900219257193&hl=en&as_sdt=6&as_vis=1&oi=scholarr

Thaler, J. (2021). The next surges are here: What can American governments lawfully do in response to the ongoing COVID-19 pandemic? *Mitchell Hamline Law Journal of Public Policy and Practice, 42*(1), 165–221. Retrieved from https://open.mitchellhamline.edu/cgi/viewcontent.cgi?article=1049&context=policypractice

Velazquez, R. (2020, July 14). Charge dropped against Chincoteague pastor suing Virginia governor. *Salisbury Daily Times*. Retrieved from https://www.delmarvanow.com/story/news/local/maryland/2020/07/14/charge-dropped-against-chincoteague-pastor-suing-virginia-governor/5437820002/

Watson, D. (2020, April 12). Holly Springs MS church goes to Walmart. *YouTube*. Retrieved from https://www.youtube.com/watch?v=2E6nqW6q4vk

Wiley, L. F., & Vladek, S. I. (2020). Coronavirus, civil liberties and the courts: The case against suspending judicial review. *Harvard Law Review, 133*(9), 179–198. Retrieved from https://harvardlawreview.org/wp-content/uploads/2020/07/179-198_Online.pdf

Chapter Four

Domestic Disjointed Narratives of the Pandemic

The Critical Early Months

Rachel Kaplan

"THE SHIFTING FRAME AND COVID-19"

Political leaders rely upon framing as a way to communicate messages to the public. Dietram Scheufele (1999) states, "Within the realm of political communication, framing has to be defined and operationalized on the basis of this social constructivism" (p. 105). Gaye Tuchman (1978) claims, "Mass media actively set the frames of reference that readers or viewers use to interpret and discuss public events" (p. ix). The mass media and political leaders tend to be the co-creators of the frames around major news stories and health crises. Arjen Bion, Paul 't Hart, and Allan McConnell (2009) indicate, "Crises thus generate framing contests to interpret events, their causes, and the responsibilities and lessons involved in ways that suit their political purposes and visions of future policy directions" (p. 81). Therefore, language creates reality for many who are consuming the media reports.

The frames associated with COVID-19 have shifted rapidly in the United States. This chapter examines mass media news reports that were about the COVID-19 crisis in the United States. Inaction in the critical early months of the pandemic set a disaster course for the pandemic in the months to come—this chapter documents mixed messages that the American public received early in the pandemic. I assert these mixed messages lead to inaction; such a documentation serves as an important lesson for future generations.

In early January 2020, the threat of COVID-19 was framed as a problem of the "other" and not a huge threat to the American public. On January 8, 2020, the CDC issued a public warning about the outbreak in China, and suggested people should take precautions when traveling to Wuhan (Blake, 2020). Greg Kelly of Newsmax interviewed Dr. Anthony Fauci on January 21, 2020, and asked, "Bottom line, we don't have to worry about this one, right?" Fauci replied,

> Well, you know, obviously we need to take it seriously and do the kinds of things that the CDC and the Department of Homeland Security are doing. But this is not a major threat for the people in the United States, and this is not something that the citizens of the United States right now should be worried about. (Kelly, 2020, 4:25–4:34)

The frame shifted once again on January 30, 2020, as Commerce Secretary Wilbur Ross suggested COVID-19 may be a good thing for the economy because it will cause businesses to re-shore their manufacturing operations. Ross stated, "I think it will help to accelerate the return of jobs to North America, some to [the] U.S., probably some to Mexico as well" (Siegel, 2020, para. 3). This frame leads the audience to believe that there may be economic prosperity because of COVID-19.

In early March 2020, President Trump told supporters at a rally in New Hampshire that the virus will go away as temperatures rise and the virus will "miraculously" go away (Beals, 2020, para. 3). In the middle of March 2020, the text in the frames shifted to concern and precaution as schools began to close, overseas travel was restricted, and Disneyland and Disney World closed (Dewan, 2020). CBS News reported on April 29, 2020,

> The U.S. coronavirus death toll topped 60,000 on Wednesday, according to Johns Hopkins University. COVID-19 has already claimed more American lives than the Vietnam War. But despite the mounting toll, more state and city leaders plan to ease restrictions aimed at curbing the virus' spread. (Reals et al., 2020, para. 1)

According to Boin, 't Hart, and McConnell (2009), "In instances where denial is no longer a credible option, debates about responsibility, blame and policy implications take a different turn depending upon which causal story about the nature and genesis of unscheduled events comes to prevail . . . " (p. 86). In the months following the March 2020 debates about blame, responsibility, and how to end the crisis dominated media channels.

In April 2020, schools remained closed, college campuses were closed, many businesses were closed, and millions of jobs have been lost. The frames constructed about COVID-19 have shifted from a problem of the other to a problem that will go away on its own to a problem that is very serious and has shut down the country. This chapter explores framing theory and three main narrative themes: COVID-19 as a problem of the other, COVID-19 is not a huge problem and will "miraculously" go away, and COVID-19 is a significant threat to America, killing large numbers of Americans. This chapter documents the transformation and evolution of the three narrative themes. The temporal dimension of the three themes begins in January 2020, when COVID-19 is not a major threat, and then shifts in March and April of 2020 as a huge threat to the USA.

Lastly, this chapter explores the implications of ever-changing news coverage and shifting rhetoric resulting in vaccine hesitancy, and documents the three shifting themes in the early months, and their implications. Also, this work documents the subsequent fallouts of these shifting themes which lays the groundwork for the discussion of Trump's COVID illness and widespread vaccine hesitancy in the USA. So, although Trump's illness and vaccine hesitancy did not happen in the early months, they represented ties/connections with the three shifting themes identified earlier and the chaos that ensued.

FRAMING THEORY

Framing theory is based upon the assumption that the media or political officials construct frames giving an event a specific meaning. In *Frame Analysis: An Essay on the Organization of Experience* (1974), Irving Goffman proposes frames provide a way to organize experiences, and frames provide people a way to form perceptions of the world around them. Frames highlight some information and leave out other bits of information. Goffman (1974) proposes the analogy of an actual picture frame, including some facts in the picture and excluding others. Robert Entman (1993) explains that frames make some ideas salient and select facts of inclusion, and that frames define problems, diagnose problems, make moral judgements, and suggest remedies. In *Frame Analysis*, Goffman (1974) develops his theory using the insights of William James, Alfred Schutz, and Gregory Bateson. Frame analysis begins by considering the very broad question, "What is it that's going on in here?" although that question can create a bias toward a unitary moment in time and may guide perspective to an event (Goffman, 1974, p. 9).

Bias is necessary for interpreting life. Goffman (1974) claims, "My aim is to try to isolate some of the basic frameworks of understanding available in our society for making sense out of events and to analyze the special vulnerabilities to which these frames of reference are subject" (p. 10). According to Goffman (1974), understanding "what is going on here" requires a firm grasp of the ideas of perspective and point of view.

Gail Fairhurst and Robert Sarr (1996) suggest that leaders can use framing techniques to create mental models for their audience, metaphors, stories, traditions, slogans, and spin. Arguably, news reporting is an exercise in creating a frame. It is important to note, "News is not a natural phenomenon emerging from facts in real life, but socially and culturally determined" (Caldas-Coulthard, 2003, p. 273).

FRAME OF "A PROBLEM OF THE OTHER"

Peter Berger and Thomas Luckman (1991) explain the world is socially constructed and language creates reality. The themes of what constitutes both knowledge and reality are explored throughout their work. The news and media are partaking in the social construction process when they report on an event. The importance of the words one chooses to explain *reality* is very important to how the audience perceives the message. Carmen Caldas-Coulthard (2003) suggests, "News therefore, has a social, a political and an educational role. By being exposed to news, people make connections and try to understand and explain how events reported in the media relate to society as a whole" (p. 273). In times of crisis, "government actors and their critics will try to escape blame for their occurrence, consolidate strengthen their political capital, and advance/defend the policies they stand for" (Boin, 't Hart, & McConnell, 2009, p. 81). The literature on blame management addresses the mechanisms determining the fate of officeholders in the wake of major disturbances and scandals (Hood et al., 2007). Caldas-Coulthard (2003) indicates, "News in the written press is a specific kind of mass media discourse which for many people enjoys a privileged and prestigious position in our culture's hierarchy of values" (p. 274).

For the purpose of this work, when the President addresses from the Oval Office and the reporting thereafter is considered news. In Western societies, people are exposed to media language probably more than any other kind of language, since its production is immense. People watch or read "news" because they think "news" is about reality (Caldas-Coulthard, 2003, p. 274). The implication is that if you are exposed to news, you are more knowledgeable about social facts (p. 274). The truth is, the news has a large element of recontextualization which involves substitution, deletion, or addition of elements. Per Linell (1998) suggests recontextualization is not a simple movement of one fixed meaning to another fixed meaning; rather, recontextualization involves transformation of meaning. Oftentimes these transformations come in the form of semantic discourse. A rhetor may choose to endorse, oppose, or "re-perspectivize" elements of a prior text, refashioning those elements as demanded by a new situation (Linell 1998, p. 151). Part of the recontextualization process involves creating and repeating metaphors. Elena Semino, Alice Deignan, and Jeannett Littlemore (2013) state, "It has also been shown that particularly prominent metaphors for specific topics can be employed in different ways in different contexts" (p. 41).

President Trump has rhetorically cast the coronavirus as a problem of the other. The president has employed the phrase the "Chinese Virus" to imply otherness. Trump attempted to create the illusion that this virus is a foreign problem. On March 11, 2020, President Trump addressed the nation from the Oval Office, and he stressed the importance of banning all travel from China to the United States on January 31, 2020, and on March 11, 2020, he implemented a ban of travel from all European nations (White House, 2020). In this same address, the President stated that young and healthy people will recover from the virus, and it is the elderly that needs to be concerned. These sentiments also put forth the illusion that this was a virus for only the elderly to worry about. Calling the coronavirus the Chinese Virus was intentional. An article in the *Washington Post* reported photos taken by Jabin Botsford to show Trump deliberately crossing out the word "Corona" on his speech notes in March 2020 and replacing it with the word "Chinese" (Botsford, 2020, picture #5; Chiu, 2020).

According to the website Factbase the President used the expression "Chinese Virus" more than 20 times between March 16, 2020 and March 30, 2020 (Viala-Gaudefroy & Lindaman, 2020, para. 3). It appears that the term "Chinese Virus" has sparked increased racist acts and hate crimes against Chinese Americans. The *New York Times* reported about a twenty-six-year-old woman from China who has lived in San Francisco for five years; she was spit on and shouted at on her way to the gym in March. Tony Du, an epidemiologist in Howard County, Maryland, who fears for his son, Larry, said, "If they keep using these terms, the kids are going to pick it up. . . . They are going to call my 8-year-old son a Chinese virus. It's serious" (Tavernise & Oppell, 2020, para. 9). *PBS NewsHour* also reported several hate crimes against Chinese Americans; one man was coughed on and shouted at in a grocery store line, and Jeni Erbes-Chan, an architect in New York, was insulted on a trip in the subway on March 10th, 2020 (Loffman, 2020). Erbes-Chan said, "A man sort of lurched at me and shouted, 'You people brought the virus. Go back to China.' I was a little in shock . . . " (para. 5). These types of anti-Chinese hate incidents were reported on mainstream media outlets. The idea that the coronavirus was an Asian problem created a scapegoat frame.

SCAPEGOATING

A common response to economic or political distress is to seek to "apportion blame" (Gibson & Howard, 2007, p. 193). Scapegoating appears to be used in the narrative creation process when making the coronavirus a problem of the other. Scapegoating shifts the focus from what is actually occurring to who is to blame for the problem. Scapegoating is dangerous and can be a contributing factor in hate crimes. James Gibson and Marc Howard (2007) assert that Scapegoat theory has long been utilized to justify and explain outbreaks of intolerance and repression of minority groups, and explain that "[t]he process is simple: when there is tension and social problems seem insurmountable, find an innocent, weak, and distinctive group to blame and victimize" (p. 194).

Historically, the term *scapegoating* is from the Hebrew word *Sa'ir La-'aza'zel*, and the literal translation to English is "goat for Azazel" (*Encyclopedia Britannica*, 2012). In the Old Testament, Azazel is a demon-like character; the goat was burdened with the sins of the Jewish people. The slaughter of the goat was a source of relief of sin and atonement for the sins of the Jewish people. William Tyndale created the English word *scapegoat* in 1530 (Holloway, 2019). Tyndale was a Protestant scholar, and when he completed the first translation of the entire Hebrew Bible to English, he found he needed to introduce some new words into the English language in order to make sense of Hebrew (Holloway, 2019). Holloway (2019) explains,

> Today, the rituals of Yom Kippur have changed hugely since it was first described in the Torah, but the habit of blaming others for things that we ourselves have done has not changed so much since Tyndale first described it. (para. 7)

Scapegoating in times of crisis is nothing new. Scapegoating is widespread, and it can generate hate against a myriad of victims. Michael O'Flynn, Lee Monaghan, and Martin Power (2014) write about the multiple groups who were scapegoated in the aftermath of the financial crisis of 2008. They note, the scapegoating frame included "'we who went a bit mad with borrowing' to more specific groups such as public sector workers, the unemployed, single mothers and immigrants" (p. 921). Sonia Shah (2020) writes,

> . . . in 1832, a group of Irish immigrants, irrationally scorned as carriers of Cholera, were first quarantined, and then secretly massacred and buried in a mass grave. Erroneously blamed for spreading HIV in the early 1980s, Haitians were beaten and harassed. Falsely scapegoated as carriers of SARS in 2003, Canadians of Chinese descent were kicked out of their homes and their businesses avoided. (para. 3)

Scapegoating makes those in power seem like they do not have any culpability in the problem. "Othering is an omnipresent phenomenon" and the scapegoating process brings about feelings of mistrust and xenophobia (Petersson, 2003, p. 85). Scapegoating is relevant because it appears many people were blaming Chinese people for the COVID-19 virus and were scapegoating the blame on Chinese American citizens. This is evidenced with a spike in Asian American hate crimes in the United States (Chiu, 2020; Loffman, 2020).

THE FRAME OF "NOT A HUGE THREAT TO AMERICA"

In May 2018, the administration disbanded the White House Pandemic Team. As a matter of fact,

> the top White House official responsible for leading the U.S. response in the event of a deadly pandemic left the administration, and the global health security team he oversaw has been disbanded under a reorganization by national security adviser John Bolton. (Sun, 2018, para. 1)

This action left the United States in a precarious position regarding health outbreaks and threats of bioterrorism.

The sense of threat and uncertainty that crises or disasters induce "may profoundly impact people's understanding of the world around them" (Boin, 't Hart, & McConnell, 2009, p. 81). The rhetorical frame of this is "not a huge threat to America" and "The United States Government Has It Under Control" were constructed and profoundly impacted citizens' perception of the threat of the coronavirus. Jamieson and Albarracin found, "Nearly one in five of our respondents (19%) reported believing that some in the CDC are exaggerating the seriousness of the virus to undermine the Trump presidency" (2020, p. 3). The belief that the CDC (Centers for Disease Control) was exaggerating led to more people willingly and openly ignoring CDC guidance regarding masks, distancing, and adherence to other mitigation efforts.

Another media and political frame employed that seemed to minimize the threat was the necessity of mask wearing. The frame seemed to shift as to who needed a mask and when one should wear a mask. Early in the outbreak the message was clear: do not wear a mask. Elisabeth Buchwald (2020) states,

> Though health officials have warned Americans to prepare for the spread of the novel coronavirus in the U.S., people shouldn't wear face masks to prevent the spread of the infectious illness, according to the Centers for Disease Control and Prevention, the U.S. Department of Health and Human Services and the U.S. surgeon general. (para. 1)

Johns Hopkins University reports that there was a clear and delineated shift in the rhetoric regarding the wearing of masks. In early April 2020, the Centers for Disease Control and Prevention revised its guidance to recommend that in addition to social distancing measures, all Americans should wear masks when leaving the house (*Hub* Staff, 2020). President Donald Trump addressed the nation on April 3rd, 2020, explaining that the CDC issued a recommendation that all Americans should wear a mask when leaving their home (Associated Press, 2020). In his closing remarks to the nation Trump said, "I just don't . . . I don't know, somehow I don't see it for myself" (Rev, 2020, 29:21). This comment denotes a clear shift in presidential rhetoric as Donald Trump publicly stated he was choosing to disregard the CDC's recommendation. I believe this created a pivotal moment in mass media coverage as the Presidential address was broadcasted to homes all across the country. This public disregard of masks and the need for masking in public left citizens questioning if they should follow the President or the CDC.

Associate Professor Kirsten Koehler, of the Department of Environmental Health and Engineering at the Bloomberg School of Public Health, explained the shift in rhetoric was partly due to the virus spreading among asymptomatic carriers of COVID-19 (*Hub* Staff, 2020). People may be carriers of the virus but not show any symptoms; therefore, wearing a mask serves as a way to protect others from their respiratory droplets.

Mask mandates were occurring all over the country, and each state, county, and municipality seemed to make their own rules regarding when and if one needed to wear a mask. Masks became a symbol of one taking responsibility for their health and the health of their community, and masks became a political symbol. Elena Schneider (2020) indicates, "President Donald Trump's reluctance to embrace masks during the coronavirus pandemic has turned them into a political object despite his own administration's public health advice" (para. 1). Mask wearing became a partisan issue. Nick Everhart, a Republican ad-maker, commented about masks and their place in political advertisements,

> The amount of mask-wearing in TV ads often aligns with the partisan index of the district and how deeply, or not, the district has dealt with coronavirus. . . . Certainly, in the current political moment, [an ad] with or without a mask . . . can send a lot of signals and messages. (Schneider, 2020, para. 6)

President Donald Trump hosted mask-less rallies and packed people into crowded spaces to launch his reelection campaign. His rallies occurred all across the United States. For example, on September 10, 2020, in Freeland, Michigan over four thousand people crowded into a hangar space and some flowed outside, and only a minority of people wore masks. In September

2020 thousands of supporters rallied for Trump in a warehouse at Henderson, Nevada. *USA Today* reported that, "he [Trump] didn't just defy state orders and federal health guidelines. He left a trail of coronavirus outbreaks in his wake" (Mansfield, Salman, & Pulver, 2020, para. 1). *USA Today* conducted an analysis to determine the trend of cases that occurred in areas of the country where people attended the rallies. Mansfield and associates (2020) report, "A *USA TODAY* analysis shows COVID-19 cases grew at a faster rate than before after at least five of those rallies in the following counties: Blue Earth, Minnesota; Lackawanna, Pennsylvania; Marathon, Wisconsin; Dauphin, Pennsylvania; and Beltrami, Minnesota" (para. 2). Dr. Fauci alarms,

> It doesn't matter who you are or where you are, when you have congregate settings where people are crowded together and virtually no one is wearing a mask, that's a perfect setup to have an outbreak of acquisition and transmissibility. . . . (Riechmann, 2020, para. 4)

Rhetorically, President Trump took the stance that masks were a personal choice and should not be forced by a government agency. Masking is still a point of contention and many Americans are expressing that they are unwilling to mask. President Trump refused to wear a mask at his rallies. The president, at the age of seventy-four, and the first lady tested positive for COVID-19 on October 2, 2020 (Vox, 2020). President Trump was treated at the Walter Reed National Military Medical Center in Washington and released on October 5, 2020. Trump was treated with antiviral Remdesivir (Belluz, 2020). President Trump framed the illness as "no big deal" through his actions. He did not isolate for the full ten days recommended by the CDC, and instead,

> he rode in a car with others on day four of his symptoms, and on day five, took off his mask as he entered the White House. As of Wednesday, he'd returned to the Oval Office to work—necessitating those around him to don N95 masks, gowns, and gloves. (Belluz, 2020, para. 8)

These actions frame the infectious disease COVID-19 as "not that big of a deal" when in fact hundreds of thousands of American citizens died as a result of COVID-19.

VACCINE HESITANCY NARRATIVE

In 2017, about three years before the COVID-19 pandemic started in the United States, the *Journal of the American Medicinal Association* published an article citing concerns about the Trump administration spreading vaccine narratives that encourage vaccine hesitancy (Sharfstein, 2017). The article cites three different concerns about the Trump administration in regard to vaccines. The first concern was that there will likely be greater attention to theories that vaccines cause harm, and this could be through the presidential comments erroneously linking autism and vaccines or tweets from high-ranking officials (Sharfstein, 2017). The second perceived foreseeable challenge to vaccination was based on the individualist ideology that individual rights are more important than the greater good, and the government should not tell people what to do. The third concern was the potential to undermine science, specifically undermine trust in our nation's system that generates and evaluates evidence (Sharfstein, 2017). Vaccine hesitancy and distrust of vaccine science were omnipresent bipartisan concerns cited in a letter constructed by Senate and House leaders in 2017 (Sharfstein, 2017).

Despite the concerns noted by President Trump in 2017 regarding vaccines, in the midst of the Covid-19 pandemic he and his team developed Operation Warp Speed aimed at producing vaccines capable of preventing COVID-19. Moncef Slaoui and Matthew Hepburn (2020) state,

> Announced on May 15, Operation Warp Speed (OWS)—a partnership of the Department of Health and Human Services (HHS), the Department of Defense (DOD), and the private sector—aims to accelerate control of the Covid-19 pandemic by advancing development, manufacturing, and distribution of vaccines, therapeutics, and diagnostics. (2020, p. 1701)

The vaccine was released in December 2020 and brought great relief to some people while others viewed the vaccine as a fake panacea.

According to the *Bloomberg* COVID-19 vaccine tracker, as of August 1, 2021, in the U.S., 346 million doses had been given. In October 2021, an average of one million doses per day were administered (Vaccine Tracker, 2021). Though 65.3 percent of people were vaccinated with at least one dose and 56.4 percent are fully vaccinated in the United States, 34.7 percent of people were not (Vaccine Tracker, 2021, October 10). There are numerous reasons people provide why they are hesitant to receive the vaccine. G. Troiano and A. Nardi (2021) explain,

> The most given reasons to refuse vaccine were as follows: being against vaccines in general, concerns about safety/thinking that a vaccine produced in a rush is too dangerous, considering the vaccine useless because of the harmless nature of COVID-19, general lack of trust, doubts about the efficiency of the vaccine, belief to be already immunized, doubt about the provenience of vaccine. (p. 245)

There is a lot of vaccine hesitancy in the United States, contributing to the spread of COVID-19 and variants of COVID-19. Some of these events, especially the COVID-19 vaccine release in December 2020, should not be considered a part of the "early months" of the COVID-19 pandemic. However, I do argue there are implications of the shifting and inconsistent rhetorical positions presented to the American public regarding vaccine science from the pre-pandemic era that have framed vaccines in general in a negative way. Hence, it should not come as a surprise that the COVID-19 vaccine is being met with skepticism and resistance.

CONCLUSION

Goffman (1974) asserts that framing theory allows a way for one to sort through a complex situation and answer the question, "What is going on here?" Frames provide an arbitrary starting and ending point to a crisis and allow some facts to become salient and other points to become invisible. This work highlighted three main themes: COVID-19 seems to be a problem of the other; COVID-19 is not a significant problem and will "miraculously" go away; and COVID-19 is a huge threat to America, killing large numbers of Americans. Constructing these themes is an act of framing, and these frames highlight the Federal government's response to the COVID-19 crisis and the mainstream media's reporting of numerous events. These events include the slow and inconsistent masking recommendations offered by the Federal government, President Trump hosting large public mask-less rallies, and the inconsistent messaging regarding vaccine science.

This work documents the transformation and evolution of the three narrative themes. The temporal dimension of the three themes begins in January 2020, when COVID-19 is not a major threat, and then shifts in March and April of 2020 as a significant threat to the United States, and lastly this chapter explores the implications of ever-changing news coverage and rhetorical bias in July of 2021 resulting in vaccine hesitancy. The historical moment we are living through is relevant when considering framing of the COVID-19 pandemic.

Ronald Arnett, Janie Fritz, and Leeanne Bell (2009) explain we are living in Postmodernity in which difference and narrative disagreement define the time period. The mere construct of difference defines our daily existence, and this is brought to the forefront with the differing narratives of the COVID-19 pandemic. Arnett, Fritz, and Bell (2009) note that as a society we do not agree on what values or the general good we will choose to protect and promote, and narrative disagreement is showcased through a clashing of political opinions and debates on ethics and morals.

Society members do not subscribe to the same narrative ground regarding what constitutes what is right and what is wrong. The COVID-19 pandemic highlighted the difference in this nation. Some people found masks to be an intrusion on their personal freedom, while others found comfort in masks to be a scientifically proven way to decrease the spread of respiratory droplets. Some people chose to socially distance themselves from their friends and family to protect themselves and their communities, while others continued to gather. Some people rushed for the COVID-19 vaccines, while others refused it. Framing theory influences people, and people rely on frames to make decisions. The salience of different facts varies and is clearly seen when reflecting upon the behaviors of different people.

The aforementioned research led to some generalized conclusions. The United States was not prepared at all for the pandemic: the national stockpile of masks was insufficient; we lacked a pandemic response team, and, due to the erroneous optimistic frame, it led to high death tolls; the continuous lack of a national policy; and states that adopted inaction ended up as hot spots in the pandemic.

REFERENCES

Arnett, R. C., Fritz, J. M. H., & Bell, L. M. (2009). *Communication ethics: Literacy dialogue and difference*. Los Angeles: Sage Publications.

Associated Press. (2020, April 3). Trump on mask wearing: "I don't think" I'll do it. [Video]. *New York Times.* Retrieved from https://www.nytimes.com/video/us/politics/100000007070943/trump-mask-coronavirus.html

Blake, A. (2020, April 21). Analysis | 2 months in the dark: The increasingly damning timeline of Trump's coronavirus response. *The Washington Post*. Retrieved from https://www.washingtonpost.com/politics/2020/04/07/timeline-trumps-coronavirus-response-is-increasingly-damning/

Beals, R. K. (2020, March 16). Trump believes coronavirus will vanish with April temps—experts are skeptical warm weather alone is enough: COVID-19 advances the tough dialogue about climate change and contagion. *MarketWatch*. Retrieved from https://www.marketwatch.com/story/trump-believes-coronavirus-will-vanish-with-april-temps-experts-are-skeptical-warm-weather-alone-is-enough-2020-03-12

Belluz, J. (2020, October 8). Trump returned to the Oval Office. He may still be contagious. *Vox*. Retrieved from https://www.vox.com/2020/10/7/21503932/trump-coronavirus-contagious-covid-19

Berger, P. L., & Luckmann, T. (1991). *The social construction of reality: A treatise in the sociology of knowledge* (10th ed.). London, UK: Penguin.

Boin, A., Hart, P., & McConnell, A. (2009). Crisis exploitation: Political and policy impacts of framing contests. *Journal of European Public Policy, 16*(1), 81–106. Retrieved from https://doi.org/10.1080/13501760802453221

Botsford, J. (2020, December 29). President Trump's tumultuous 2020: A look at President Trump's most consequential year. *The Washington Post*. Retrieved from https://www.washingtonpost.com/graphics/politics/2020/12/29/president-trumps-tumultuous-2020/?itid=ap_jabinbotsford

Buchwald, E. (2020, March 2). U.S. health officials say Americans shouldn't wear face masks to prevent coronavirus—here are 3 other reasons not to wear them. *MarketWatch*. Retrieved from https://www.marketwatch.com/story/the-cdc-says-americans-dont-have-to-wear-facemasks-because-of-coronavirus-2020-01-30

Caldas-Coulthard, C. R. (2003). Cross-cultural representation of "otherness" in media discourse. In G. Weiss & R. Wodak (Eds.), *Critical discourse analysis: Theory and disciplinarity* (pp. 272–296). London, UK: Palgrave Macmillan.

Chiu, A. (2020, March 20). Trump has no qualms about calling coronavirus the "Chinese Virus." That's a dangerous attitude, experts say. *The Washington Post*. Retrieved from https://www.washingtonpost.com/nation/2020/03/20/coronavirus-trump-chinese-virus/.

Dewan, A. (2020, March 13). The US is starting to look like Italy on coronavirus lockdown. It could learn a thing or two. Retrieved from https://www.cnn.com/2020/03/13/americas/coronavirus-us-italy-south-korea-lessons-intl/index.html

Entman, R. M. (1993). Framing: Toward clarification of a fractured paradigm. *Journal of Communication, 43*(4), 51–58. Retrieved from https://doi.org/10.1111/j.1460-2466.1993.tb01304.x

Fairhurst, G., & Sarr, R. (1996). *The art of framing*. San Francisco: Jossey-Bass.

Gibson, J., & Howard, M. (2007). Russian anti-Semitism and the scapegoating of Jews. *British Journal of Political Science, 37*(2), 193–223. Retrieved from https://doi.org/10.1017/S0007123407000105

Goffman, E. (1974). *Frame analysis: An essay on the organization of experience*. London: Harper and Row.

Holloway, S. (2019, October 8). The origins of the "scapegoat." *Sydney Jewish Museum*. Retrieved from https://sydneyjewishmuseum.com.au/jewish-culture/the-origins-of-the-scapegoat/#:~:text=A%20key%20part%20of%20Yom,upon%20it%2C%20would%20be%20thrown

Hood, C., Jennings, W., Hogwood, B., & Beeston, C. (2007). Fighting fires in testing times: Exploring a staged response hypothesis for blame management in two exam fiasco cases. [CARR Discussion Paper: DP 42]. *London: Centre for Analysis of Risk and Regulation, London School of Economics and Political Science*. Retrieved from http://eprints.lse.ac.uk/36122/1/Disspaper42.pdf

Hub Staff. (2020, April 24). Understanding changing guidance on mask use. *The Hub, Johns Hopkins University*. Retrieved from https://hub.jhu.edu/2020/04/24/covid-19-mask-glove-use/

Jamieson, K. H., & Albarracín, D. (2020, April 20). The relation between media consumption and misinformation at the outset of the SARS-CoV-2 pandemic in the US. *Harvard Kennedy School Misinformation Review*. Retrieved from https://

doi.org/10.37016/mr-2020-012; https://misinforeview.hks.harvard.edu/wp-content/uploads/2020/04/April19_FORMATTED_COVID-19-Survey.pdf

Kelly, G. (2020, April 6). Dr. Anthony Fauci's thoughts on COVID-19 from January 2020. *Twitter Media Studio.* Newsmax on Twitter. Retrieved from https://twitter.com/newsmax/status/1247180304823062529?lang=en

Linell, P. (1998). *Approaching dialogue: Talk, interaction and contexts in dialogical perspectives*. Amsterdam: John Benjamins Publishing.

Loffman, M. (2020, April 7). Asian Americans describe "gut punch" of racist attacks during coronavirus pandemic. *PBS NewsHour*. Retrieved from https://www.pbs.org/newshour/nation/asian-americans-describe-gut-punch-of-racist-attacks-during-coronavirus-pandemic

Mansfield, E., Salman, J., & Pulver, D. V. (2021, January 28). Trump's campaign made stops nationwide. Coronavirus cases surged in his wake in at least five places. *USA Today*. Retrieved from https://www.usatoday.com/story/news/investigations/2020/10/22/trumps-campaign-made-stops-nationwide-then-coronavirus-cases-surged/3679534001/

O'Flynn, M., Monaghan, L. F., & Power, M. J. (2014). Scapegoating during a time of crisis: A critique of post-Celtic Tiger Ireland. *Sociology*, *48*(5). 921–937. Doi:10.1177/0038038514539059

Petersson, B. (2003). Combating uncertainty, combating the global: scapegoating, xenophobia and the national-local nexus. *International Journal of Peace Studies, 8*(1), 85–102. Retrieved from https://www.jstor.org/stable/41852895

Reals, T., McNamara, A., Carissimo, J., & Pawlikowski, J. (2020, April 30). Coronavirus updates from April 29, 2020. *CBS News*. Retrieved from https://www.cbsnews.com/live-updates/coronavirus-live-updates-2020-04-29/

Rev. (2020, April 3). Donald Trump coronavirus briefing transcript April 3: New CDC face mask recommendation [Video transcript]. *Rev Transcripts*. Retrieved from https://www.rev.com/blog/transcripts/donald-trump-coronavirus-briefing-transcript-april-3-new-cdc-face-mask-recommendations

Riechmann, D. (2020, October 29). As virus surges, Trump rallies keep packing in thousands. *AP NEWS*. Retrieved from https://apnews.com/article/donald-trump-rallies-virus-surges-50e79fabd46472c51ecc1444184082de

Scheufele, D. A. (1999). Framing as a theory of media effects. *Journal of Communication*, *49*(1), 103–122. Retrieved from https://doi.org/10.1111/j.1460-2466.1999.tb02784.x

Schneider, E. (2020, September 30). The face mask "is almost as much of a symbol as a MAGA hat." *POLITICO*. Retrieved from https://www.politico.com/news/2020/09/30/face-masks-political-ads-coronavirus-424149

Semino, E., Deignan, A., & Littlemore, J. (2013). Metaphor, genre, and recontextualization. *Metaphor and Symbol*, *28*(1), 41–59. Retrieved from https://doi.org/10.1080/10926488.2013.742842

Shah, S. (2020, March 7). The pandemic of xenophobia and scapegoating. *Time*. Retrieved from https://time.com/5776279/pandemic-xenophobia-scapegoating/

Sharfstein, J. M. (2017). Vaccines and the Trump administration. *Jama*, *317*(13), 1305–1306. doi:10.1001/jama.2017.2311

Siegel, R. (2020, January 30). Commerce Secretary Wilbur Ross says China's coronavirus "will help" bring jobs back to U.S. *The Washington Post*. Retrieved from https://www.washingtonpost.com/business/2020/01/30/wilbur-ross-coronavirus-jobs

Slaoui, M., & Hepburn, M. (2020). Developing safe and effective Covid vaccines—Operation Warp Speed's strategy and approach. *New England Journal of Medicine*, *383*(18), 1701–1703. Doi:10.1056/NEJMp2027405

Sun, L. (2018, May 10). Top White House official in charge of pandemic response exits abruptly. *Washington Post*. Retrieved from https://www.washingtonpost.com/news/to-your-health/wp/2018/05/10/top-white-house-official-in-charge-of-pandemic-response-exits-abruptly/

Tavernise, S., & Oppel, R. (2020, March 23). Spit on, yelled at, attacked: Chinese-Americans fear for their safety. *New York Times*. Retrieved from https://www.nytimes.com/2020/03/23/us/chinese-coronavirus-racist-attacks.html

The Editors of *Encyclopedia Britannica*. (2012, August 6). Scapegoat. *Britannica.com*. Retrieved from https://www.britannica.com/topic/scapegoat

The White House. (2020, March 11). President Trump addresses the nation on COVID-19: Get the latest information from the CDC about COVID-19. [Trump White House Archived Video, WH.gov]. *YouTube*. Retrieved from https://www.youtube.com/watch?v=6a1Mdq8-_wo

Troiano, G., & Nardi, A. (2021). Vaccine hesitancy in the era of COVID-19. *PubMed Central*, May (194), 245–251. doi:101.1016/j/puhe/2021.02.025.

Tuchman, G. (1978). *Making news: A study in the construction of reality*. New York: Free Press.

Vaccine Tracker [updated]. (2021, October 10). More than 6.49 billion shots given: Covid-19 tracker; In the U.S., 402 million doses have been administered. *Bloomberg.com*. Retrieved from https://www.bloomberg.com/graphics/covid-vaccine-tracker-global-distribution/

Viala-Gaudefroy, J., & Lindaman, D. (2020, April 21). Donald Trump's "Chinese virus": The politics of naming. *The Conversation*. Retrieved from https://theconversation.com/donald-trumps-chinese-virus-the-politics-of-naming-136796

Vox Staff. (2020, October 2). President Trump tests positive for the coronavirus. *Vox*. Retrieved from https://www.vox.com/21498510/president-trump-covid-19-test-positive-coronavirus.

Chapter Five

Historical vs. Ahistorical Narratives of the Pandemic

The Discordant Rhetoric of Our Unprecedented Times

John J. Rief

INTRODUCTION: A DOUBLE PANDEMIC

The COVID-19 pandemic has invited numerous manifestations of discordance across social, economic, political, and ideological divides in the United States.[1] Disagreement as to the nature of the crisis, how to address it, and even its existence has undermined the development of strategies for coping with and ending the tragic pain and loss of life we have been experiencing. As I write this chapter, 5.21 million individuals, including over 790,000 in the United States, have died (Worldometer, 2021a). Why? At one level, the biological characteristics of COVID-19, especially the recently emergent Delta variant, have given it an "evolutionary edge" (Zimmer, 2021, para. 1), allowing it to spread quickly through the global population. But this alone does not account for our experience. In addition, the spread of poor information and extreme polarization in the U.S. have crafted numerous *discordant pandemic narratives,* augmenting the implications of COVID-19 far beyond what they should have been for our nation. As the communication scholar Carolyn A. Lin (2020) argued: "In the context of the current coronavirus infodemic, this politicization process has barricaded a standard scientific approach to manage the pandemic and resulted in multiple waves of rising infection rates and fatalities" (p. 667; see also, GPMB, 2020, p. 13). Indeed, ease of transmission, failed policy, poor information, and politicization have fostered a cultural, political, and ecological admixture fitted for producing high morbidity and mortality.

Furthermore, the characteristics of our public life adumbrated above have overlain a deeper pathological relationship to our past, one that has unfortunately been a feature of human communities facing disease outbreaks across time. In the preface to the newest edition of the landmark text *Epidemics and Society: From the Black Death to the Present,* published as the COVID-19 pandemic emerged, the medical historian Frank Snowden (2020) observed, "Particularly since the outburst of H5N1 influenza in 1997, the public health community has consistently sounded the alarm. Its message is that future outbreaks are inevitable" (p. x). As an example, Snowden (2020, p. xi) pointed to a crucial report by the Global Preparedness Monitoring Board (GPMB, 2019), a public health advocacy body that works in coordination with the World Health Organization (WHO) and the World Bank, entitled *A World at Risk*. This report could not have been clearer about the real and present danger of disease outbreaks on the eve of another global disaster:

> The world is at acute risk for devastating regional or global disease epidemics or pandemics that not only cause loss of life but upend economies and create social chaos.
>
> Vulnerability is heightened by an increase in outbreaks occurring in complex humanitarian emergencies, as well as a novel convergence of ecological, political, economic, and social trends including population growth, increased urbanization, a globally integrated economy, widespread and faster travel, conflict, migration and climate change. (GPMB, 2019, pp. 11–12)

Many of these same factors, including population growth, globalization, and urbanization, have been noted by classicists, historians, and public health experts as key catalysts for outbreaks going all the way back to the ancient world (Ding, 2014; Harper, 2017). Furthermore, to underscore the growing threat of pandemic disease, the report noted the frequency of disease outbreaks in recent history: "Between 2011 and 2018, WHO tracked 1483 epidemic events in 172 countries" (GPMB, 2019, p. 12). One of the report's most prescient and, in hindsight, disturbing sections is entitled "Preparing for the worst: a rapidly spreading lethal respiratory pathogen pandemic" (GPMB, 2019, p. 27). As COVID-19 was beginning its deadly march across the globe fueled by the respiratory exchange of viral particles, the GPMB was warning the international community about just this sort of pathogenic crisis.

A World at Risk warned not only of a coming pandemic but also of a cultural and political pathology that might undermine our efforts to address it:

"For too long, we have allowed a cycle of panic and neglect when it comes to pandemics: we ramp up efforts when there is a serious threat, then quickly forget about them when the threat subsides" (GPMB, 2019, p. 6). Echoing the GPMB, Snowden (2020) argued, "along with outbreaks, a recurring pattern of social amnesia has prevailed" (p. x). Indeed, one year after *A World at Risk*, the GPMB (2020) would release its follow-up report, *A World in Disorder*, which documented early efforts to address the COVID-19 pandemic. This report concluded in part that "little progress has been made on any of the actions called for in last year's report and that this lack of leadership is exacerbating the pandemic" (p. 44). The GPMB (2020) also noted the risks associated with forgetting the knowledge we have gained during the pandemic: "Failure to learn the lessons of COVID-19, or to act on them with the necessary resources and commitment, will mean that the next pandemic, which is sure to come, will be even more damaging" (p. 44). In its most recent publication, *A World Prepared*, the GPMB (2021) offered a "strategic plan" (throughout) that affirmed its commitment to advocating for historically informed pandemic, epidemic, and health crisis responses. The message is clear: failing to draw actionable knowledge from previous outbreaks leaves us constantly and consistently underprepared. COVID-19 is merely the most recent episode of a longer-term process of forgetting, of the discordance between past and present in our responses to pandemics.

The remainder of this chapter argues that it is time to recognize that we are embedded in a double pandemic. One element is rooted in a biological interaction between our immune systems and the "virosphere" (Preston, 2020, p. 372). The other is rooted in a variety of rhetorical pathologies, including the spread of poor information, entrenched politicization and polarization, and a long-established practice of forgetting.[2] It is the last of these elements, forgetting as a rhetorical maneuver and cultural practice, that frames my work. Media coverage, political rhetoric, and public health messaging about the pandemic have been thoroughly saturated by the use of the term "unprecedented." I argue that "unprecedented" is a term of ultimate discordance—a way of dividing us from our past. Thus, it renders our history unavailable as a resource to cultivate publicly useful memories. Indeed, the rhetorical effort to construct our times as unprecedented undermines sense-making and decision-making, leaving us with denuded ground upon which to understand our context and respond to it.

The following sections unpack manifestations of *the rhetoric of unprecedentedness* that have played a significant role in constructing our experiences of COVID-19. The point is to show how articulating our present as unprecedented does damage both to our collective psyches and public memories as it sows discord between our past and present. As the scholar Paula A. Treichler (1999) argued in a series of outstanding essays on the early years of HIV/

AIDS collected in *How to Have Theory in an Epidemic*, "Language is not a substitute for reality; it is one of the most significant ways we know reality, experience it, and articulate it; indeed, language plays a powerful role in producing experience and in certifying that experience as 'authentic'" (p. 4). Following Treichler's cue about the centrality of language in constructing public understandings of pandemic disease, this chapter reveals *unprecedentedness* as a "terministic screen" (Burke, 1966, p. 44) that inflects public discourse with an ahistorical framework for the evaluation of COVID-19 and our responses to it. I then invite a turn to a *rhetoric of precedence* (by which I mean a rhetoric that emphasizes the role of memory in framing contemporary action, thus drawing on an older sense of the term "precedence") as one way to frame narratives of pandemic life through the lens of history, thus bringing past and present into concordance. This rhetoric of precedence creates opportunities to discover "equipment for living" (Burke, 1973, p. 293) during these difficult times. As I describe this approach, I offer the case of Taiwan and its strategy to address the COVID-19 pandemic through the lens of precedence as an alternative way a public might deal with a crisis like this. This example allows me to build upon previous scholarly work to promote more productive rhetorical practices during pandemics and epidemics, thus reducing their overall health consequences for the U.S. and global populations (see e.g., Ding, 2014; Mitchell & McTigue, 2007).

"UNPRECEDENTEDNESS": A RHETORICAL PANDEMIC

The term "unprecedented" erects a wall between a past devoid of analogic material, a present left rudderless, and a future left entirely opaque. The *Oxford English Dictionary* (*OED*) (2021b) defined the term "unprecedented" as follows: "Having no precedent; unparalleled; never previously done, known, or experienced." Alternatively, the *OED* (2021a) observed, the term "precedent" refers to "a previous instance taken as an example or rule by which to be guided in similar cases or circumstances; an example by which a comparable subsequent act may be justified." To forward a claim of unprecedentedness, then, is to suggest there is nothing to draw upon from the past, no lesson or material that might give us a path forward. This does not imply there can be no such path. Indeed, necessity can be a catalyst for invention. As the Greek polymath and teacher Aristotle (1926a) noted in the *Rhetoric*, the point of the art is to address situations that are, in some fundamental sense, uncertain. However, while rhetoric, by definition, addresses uncertainty, the moments we encounter are almost never completely without precedent. Thus, drawing upon past experience, a key aspect of what Aristotle (1926b) called *phronesis,* or practical wisdom, is among the most effective ways to cultivate rhetoric responsiveness to their moments.

Unfortunately, a rhetoric of unprecedentedness has emerged during the COVID-19 pandemic, which has occluded the role historically rich analogical reasoning might play in our collective narratives about and responses to the pandemic. Ironically, the emergence of this rhetoric *is* precedented. As Snowden (2021a) noted in a lecture given as part of the Open Yale Course *Epidemics in Western Society Since 1600,*

> Often the press—which seems, I would argue, to suffer chronically from historical amnesia—it often treats the appearance of new infections as something unprecedented, unnatural, that never happened before. But the reality is that Charles Darwin was correct. We live in the midst of a constantly evolving microbial world in which the microbes have an inherent advantage because of the frequency of their mutations, and the extremely brief length of a microbial generation, compared with a human one. So, new diseases have always been emerging and appearing. (0:53–1:43)

The rest of this section tracks the eruption of the term "unprecedented" in public discourse about COVID-19. There is no singular text to which I can turn to adequately engage the rhetoric of unprecedentedness we have encountered during this pandemic. It is infused in the communicative and ideological air we are breathing. Thus, I am inspired by the rhetorical theorist Michael Calvin McGee's (1990) notion of the critic as a producer, rather than passive consumer, of their communicative ecology. As such, I see my task as being not only to identify and describe discrete uses of the term "unprecedented" but also to stitch together an account of its circulation from a variety of bits and pieces of our rhetorical landscape.

The term "unprecedented" reached a kind of online rhetorical peak in the United States and globally during the earliest days of the pandemic in the first half of 2020. We can find evidence of this peak with a simple search on *Google Trends* (n.d.). A graph of interest in the term "unprecedented" in U.S. searches from 2004 to the date of the search (the longest period available) generated with this platform on November 7, 2021, showed that interest reached its highest level just as the pandemic was taking off (images of graphs described here have been retained by author). Perhaps not surprisingly, the term achieved significant interest around December 2016 (with beginning and endpoints from around July 2016 to around June 2017), just after the election of Donald J. Trump as president. But interest in the term during the initial outbreak of the pandemic around March to April, 2020 (with beginning and endpoints from around February 2020 to around July 2020 and smaller peaks to the left and right on the graph) was double that of the earlier peak. Expanding the search to include global interest showed similar results (note that *Google Trends* is constantly updating, so these graphs will vary in appearance over time). Given what has already been noted about the history of disease outbreaks, this might come as a surprise. Throughout the twentieth century, we experienced numerous pandemics with major implications for health and society (e.g., the 1918 flu, polio, encephalitis lethargica, etc.). President Trump's candidacy, campaign, and early presidency were preceded by few if any analogous situations in recent memory. This provides backing for what Snowden and others have noted—we tend to be surprised by pandemics despite their historical regularity.

What's more, the increasing interest in the term demonstrated on *Google Trends* (n.d.) tracks with the COVID-19 incidence and fatality curves we have grown used to watching over the past year and a half as they precipitously rise, peak, and decline. Thus, there is a clear visual analogy connecting the two parts of our double pandemic. Both the biological and rhetorical elements grew explosively at around the same time. Of course, one could argue that at least some searches for this term might have been inquiries seeking to debunk the unprecedentedness of the pandemic. However, consider that if the term is being searched for at an increasing rate, it indicates significant circulation of the term and idea. When understood in tandem with the arguments below, the *Google Trends* (n.d.) results described here demonstrate the substantial infiltration of a rhetoric of unprecedentedness into our public consciousness and discourse.

There was a similar spike in the use of the term "unprecedented" in media coverage at around the same time. For example, in the *Access World News—Historical and Current* database by NewsBank, Inc., which includes thousands of publications, a search for the term "unprecedented" conducted on September 24, 2021, returned the following results: 169,093 in 2017, 170,064 in 2018, 169,725 in 2019, *416,787 in 2020*, and 177,763 in 2021. The results werre consistent from 2017 to 2019, but they jumped by more than twice (2.45 times higher) in 2020 when compared to 2019. Similar results can be found when limiting the search to the U.S.: 88,080 in 2017, 83,360 in 2018, 79,858 in 2019, *228,790 in 2020*, and 91,924 in 2021. Here again, the numbers were consistent until 2020, when they again jumped by more than twice (2.86 times higher) when compared to 2019. Thus, there was a major spike in the use of the term "unprecedented" during the year of COVID-19's initial global outbreak. Another search conducted on the same day for "COVID-19 and unprecedented" returned one result for 2019, 223,980 results for 2020, and 72,353 for 2021. If we limit the results to just the United States, we find a similar distribution with one result in 2019, 129,620 in 2020, and 39,503 in 2021. This means that of all the results mentioning the term "unprecedented" in this database during 2020, 53.7 percent also mentioned COVID-19. When limited to the U.S., 56.6 percent of materials in these searches mentioned both terms. Finally, of the 4,810,525 materials in this database that mentioned "COVID-19" in 2020, 223,980 or 4.6 percent also mentioned the term "unprecedented." When limited to the 2,527,800 materials that mentioned "COVID-19" in the U.S. during the same year, 129,620 or 5.1 percent also mentioned the term "unprecedented." These numbers and percentages have decreased in 2021.[3] All of the previous database results demonstrated the significant salience of the term "unprecedented" in journalistic coverage during the first year of the pandemic. Crucially, it is not clear why the occurrence of the term in these searches has decreased in 2021 (or why it does so in the *Google Trends* graph mentioned earlier). We are not on pace in 2021 to see the same final numbers as 2020 in any of the searches noted earlier. Thoughtful conjecture suggests that initial shock might inspire the use of the term, while later adaptation may make it less salient.

Of course, the "COVID-19 and unprecedented" results noted above do not indicate whether the term "unprecedented" was being applied directly to COVID-19 but rather that both words appeared in the same publication. For example, in one article from the U.S. results, Kathryn Palmer (2021a; 2021b) of the *Arizona Daily Star* referred to recent federal funding to address the economic consequences of the pandemic, as "unprecedented": "One of the major student support programs to come out of this unprecedented amount of federal funding is of course the debt forgiveness initiative [at Pima Community College]" (Palmer, 2021a, para. 2). In this case, it seems clear that the unprecedented funding was a result of the pandemic, which supports my argument that the term has often been used as a mechanism to narratively frame the world that COVID-19 has wrought. This particular use of the term also represented an ahistorical approach to understanding the crisis. Federal financial support for students, and all of society for that matter, has major precedents in the form of Franklin Delano Roosevelt's *New Deal* (1933–1939) and the *G.I. Bill of Rights* (1944). Admittedly, these programs were in response to very different calamities—the Great Depression and WWII—but they do indeed show how federal funding has been marshalled during challenging times in the past.

Moving beyond these initial efforts to capture the broad strokes of unprecedentedness in internet searches and media coverage, I now turn to several illustrative examples drawn from the arenas of medicine, public health, and politics. The first of these is a therapeutic move which is meant to respond to the mental health consequences of the pandemic. We have been told repeatedly that pandemic life is so exceptional, and it is wreaking havoc on our ability to cope. As the American Psychological Association (APA) (2020) reported in their *Stress in America 2020: A National Mental Health Crisis*, mental health problems are significant sequelae of the ongoing COVID-19 pandemic. This report was based on an annual survey conducted by the APA that found: "Americans have been profoundly affected by the COVID-19 pandemic, and that the external factors Americans have listed in previous years as significant sources of stress remain present and problematic" (APA, 2020, p. 1). It went on to argue that "it is the unusual combination of these factors and the persistent drumbeat of a crisis that shows no sign of abating that is leading APA to sound the alarm" (p. 1). I fundamentally agree with the APA's assessment here, especially that there is a loud "drumbeat" of unmitigated crisis, its percussive reverberations infiltrating every layer of public life.

However, I take issue with how the report narratively framed the problem and its solutions through a lens that left little sense of previous knowledge, experience, and memories as resources for overcoming the mental health consequences of the pandemic. First, the report compared the death toll of the pandemic (at the time well over two hundred thousand) to previous wars involving the U.S. (WWI, Vietnam, and Korea). This suggested that the important analogue was overall deaths as opposed to similar circumstances, for instance, the 1918 flu pandemic, which would be a much more apposite comparison. It then went on to suggest that Generation Z is "facing unprecedented uncertainty" (APA, 2020, p. 1) related not only to illness but also socio-economic and educational stressors wrought by social distancing, virtual work and learning, and the like. All of this may be true for Generation Z, but the report offered no recourse to public experiences and memories of past events that might give them an interpretive foothold. In a later section on Generation Z, the report noted: "While older Americans may be able to embrace the feeling of 'this too shall pass,' Gen Z adults (ages 18–23) are at a pivotal moment in their lives experiencing adulthood at a time when the future looks uncertain" (APA, 2020, p. 3). "This too shall pass" is an axiom rooted in historical understanding and public memories of past crises. The fact that older generations may be able to see the truth in this statement due to their past experiences provides one potential explanation for the much higher stress levels the APA found among Generation Z respondents. Perhaps a missing link for Generation Z is a narrative framing of the present rooted in life experiences, of older generations made available through robust modes of intergenerational sharing.

Finally, the APA report argued: "One of the key ways to maintain strong mental health in times of adversity is by remaining hopeful—something that a majority of Americans report, despite the compounding stress and negative impacts of the pandemic and other issues" (APA, 2020, p. 9). Indeed! However, the report did not offer a historically grounded account of how this hope might be maintained as we move forward. Fulfilling the goal set out at the beginning of the report to assist everyone to "emerge from this time in our history poised to embrace and shape a brighter future together" (APA, 2020, p. 1) requires more than psychological tools. Hope is founded on experiential narratives that provide a reason to hope, a way of making sense of why we should be hopeful. Instead of framing the pandemic's consequences as "unprecedented" and the mental health landscape as a crisis, we may find it more helpful to focus on how previous generations have survived and thrived even in trying times.

To be clear, making space to acknowledge that we all have been impacted psychically, socially, and culturally by the pandemic is important. There is a long history of ignoring mental health problems that emerge from crisis situations, a history that we must overcome. Simone Biles's recent withdrawal from competition at the 2021 Tokyo Olympics has become a landmark case of a major public figure framing mental health as a legitimate concern (Park, 2021a; 2021b). On the other hand, suggesting that our times are so exceptional that we should expect to be psychically harmed by them can invite a wholly different response. In essence, we are being told that pandemics like this, their socio-economic and other consequences, and the sacrifices we are being asked to make will lead to pathological consequences for us. While the APA report had many pieces of advice for how to become an "agent" in one's own mental health during such times, the "scene" it painted lacked crucial historical texture to generate additional *equipment for hoping* (Burke, 1952, 1973).

Another more recent feature of the rhetorical pandemic of unprecedentedness has been the conversation about the Food & Drug Administration's efforts to review and approve new vaccines for COVID-19. The speed of these efforts has often been described as "unprecedented." For instance, on its answers page for questions about the vaccines, the CDC (2021) argued:

> The federal government has worked since the start of the pandemic to make COVID-19 vaccines available as soon as possible. This accelerated timeline is unprecedented. Some people are concerned that vaccine safety may have been sacrificed in favor of speed. However, as with all vaccines, safety is a top priority in the United States and globally. (para. 1)

Moreover, in an *ABC News* article about the recent full approval of the Pfizer vaccine, Janet Woodcock, the FDA commissioner, was quoted as saying:

> Working around the clock, FDA staff were able to complete the evaluation of this biologics license application in just over three months. . . . This is an unprecedented timeline given the volume of review and the meticulous manner in which it was done, but we want to underscore that our efforts to move as quickly as possible have in no way sacrifice[d] scientific standards for the integrity of our process. (Pezenik, 2021, para. 10)

In both cases, the reader should note the emphasis placed on scientific rigor. This may have been an effort to assuage safety concerns and decrease vaccine hesitancy. Finally, according to an article in *The Hospitalist*, "asked to comment about the status of the FDA authorization of COVID-19 vaccines for younger children, Dr. [Anthony] Fauci described the current situation as one that 'might require some unprecedented and unique action' on the part of the FDA" (Splete, 2021, para. 11).

These are just a few examples of the term "unprecedented" circulating in the discussion about COVID-19 vaccines. There is truth to the claims being made, particularly the exceptional qualities of the vaccine development and approval process during the COVID-19 pandemic. However, this constant refrain of unprecedentedness occludes acknowledgment of an important historical parallel. During the early years of the HIV/AIDS pandemic in the 1980s and 1990s, LGBTQ+ activists fought with the government, specifically the FDA and the NIH, to accelerate and expand access to potentially helpful treatments, especially by challenging the clinical trials process (Epstein, 1995; Treichler, 1999). Their struggles both for recognizing the pandemic and expediting the discovery of effective treatments were dramatically presented in David France's (2012) award-winning documentary, *How to Survive a Plague*. As Stephen Holden (2012) noted in a review of the film in the *New York Times*: "Act Up (. . .) became the irresistible force that made seemingly immovable objects—government agencies and drug companies—give way, develop new treatments and speed them to market as the AIDS epidemic spread unchecked among the gay population" (para. 1). In this case, we have a precedent that eloquently demonstrated the failures of our nation to address health crises that are seemingly limited to marginalized communities (though we later found this was not the case with HIV/AIDS). However, when *everyone*, especially those with privilege, are perceived to be at risk, the institutional gears turn rapidly. Of course, no one should expect public institutions or individuals to address this textured history every time they discuss the process for COVID-19 vaccine approval. But the constant use of the term "unprecedented" in this context tends to erode our capacity to remember and productively activate this history. Such activation might enliven current discussions with and about communities that still lack access to healthcare and, due to legacies of exclusion and oppression, also and with good reason, lack trust in the healthcare industry and government.

Furthermore, the term "unprecedented" has also circulated in the political world. For example, in his first major address just after the WHO declared COVID-19 a pandemic, President Trump (2020) invoked the term "unprecedented" to describe his administration's public health measures: "My fellow Americans, tonight I want to speak with you about our nation's unprecedented response to the coronavirus outbreak that started in China and is now spreading throughout the world" (para. 1). He also used the term in the context of economic measures related to the pandemic: "I will soon be taking emergency action, which is unprecedented, to provide financial relief. This will be targeted for workers who are ill, quarantined, or caring for others due to coronavirus" (para. 22). I will not make the case that Trump was somehow "patient zero" for the rhetorical pandemic of unprecedentedness, but his moves here and throughout the rest of his speech represented many inflections of the term and its rhetorical consequences. Thus, they deserve serious attention, especially given that this speech was one of the earliest efforts to provide a national narrative framework for the pandemic.

From what we have learned of Trump, his opening statement in this speech about public health measures (the first quotation above) may have been more about establishing his leadership credibility (which waned at best and was nonexistent or counterproductive at worst) than it was about any effort to advance an ahistorical perspective on the pandemic. But it also indicated a trajectory of thinking that has been prevalent during the pandemic: the public health and economic interventions that have been implemented do not have historical parallels. Moreover, his primary discussion of history in the speech is itself noteworthy as it was so abstract it bordered on meaningless:

> From the beginning of time, nations and people have faced unforeseen challenges, including large-scale and very dangerous health threats. This is the way it always was and always will be. It only matters how you respond, and we are responding with great speed and professionalism. (Trump, 2020, para. 5)

Trump's approach to history here was largely without meaningful content and entirely unhelpful. He compounded these problems by invoking an ahistorical version of American exceptionalism:

> No nation is more prepared or more resilient than the United States. We have the best economy, the most advanced health care, and the most talented doctors, scientists, and researchers anywhere in the world. We are all in this together. We must put politics aside, stop the partisanship and unify together as one nation and one family. As history has proven time and time again, Americans always rise to the challenge and overcome adversity. (Trump, 2020, paras. 32–34)

Here we can see Trump's superficial understanding of the American progress narrative which was invoked unproblematically to suggest victory against COVID-19 was inevitable. This stance is belied by our failure to end, for instance, the HIV/AIDS epidemic or eradicate other diseases (Snowden, 2020). Trump also argued for a status quo that was largely a construction of his own mind and political rhetoric. Our economic and health care systems have not been as resilient and effective as he suggested they would be in this speech. Moreover, as with all of his attempts to argue for unity, this one faltered, especially given some of the other arguments made in the speech (see below).

Trump also listed numerous decisions his administration made, including travel restrictions impacting China and Europe, efforts to reduce or eliminate costs for COVID-19 treatments, ramping up the financial support for and speed of research into treatments (including vaccines), social distancing, and institutional closures. All these measures have past precedent, and some have been more effective than others (Snowden, 2020). The problem with framing them as somehow unprecedented is that they may have come across as overly draconian, without evidence, or unnecessary, especially given his claim that for

> the vast majority of Americans: The risk is very, very low. Young and healthy people can expect to recover fully and quickly if they should get the virus. The highest risk is for elderly population with underlying health conditions. The elderly population must be very, very careful. (Trump, 2020, para. 16)

Suggesting the need for unprecedented health measures while at the same time arguing most individuals will never have to worry about the pandemic allowed the audience to view them as draconian. It also divided the population into safe and at-risk groups. Put another way, while this passage may be read merely as an effort to assuage growing fear and anxiety by limiting the scope of risk, it also invited us/them thinking. Admittedly, Trump (2020) did state later in the speech that "each of us has a role to play in defeating this virus" (para. 21). He also listed various hygienic activities everyone could take to reduce the risk of transmission and noted policies he would implement to help people isolate and take care of themselves. But these elements ring somewhat hollow given the earlier framing. Unfortunately, this rhetorical move to divide risk between different groups broke out in conservative circles as a tool to undermine public health measures and place the onus for dealing with the pandemic on at-risk groups. For example, the Lieutenant Governor of Texas, Dan Patrick, argued that some elderly individuals would (and by implication, perhaps should) sacrifice their health and survival to rescue the economy from the ill-effects of public health measures (Knodel, 2020). Such logic does not invite unity but rather victim-blaming and scapegoating.

On the face of it, Trump's speech was an effort to show just how effective the administration had been in taking fast and efficient action while also suggesting the pandemic would be short-lived and low impact (all arguments the administration would continue to spin throughout the early days of the pandemic). But, stitching together his invocation of the term "unprecedented," his largely ahistorical framing of the public health interventions he implemented, and his argument that most Americans would not be severely impacted by COVID-19 demonstrates Trump's rhetorical stance was more complicated than it might seem. What we know of his actions following this speech and throughout the pandemic is that he was largely opposed to many public health measures, backed treatments that were ineffective or unproven, and tended to deny the depth and tragedy of the ongoing threat of COVID-19. In short, his lack of leadership during the pandemic may have been the most unprecedented element of it.

Given the broad circulation of the term "unprecedented" during the pandemic in various contexts and with different purposes as documented on the previous pages, efforts to reconnect our health communication, political rhetoric, and community discussions of COVID-19 to historical analogues and narratives gain added purchase. While there is value in recognizing the textured differences between historical and contemporary experiences with human disease, especially to deal with any new dynamics we face, taking it to the level of incommensurability undermines reflective actions with clear rationales. What's more, we have a rich past of addressing pandemics in this country, in particular the efforts undertaken by Jonas Salk and Albert Sabin to create effective vaccines for polio (Snowden, 2020). As a civilization, we have faced down many pandemics with public health measures, medicines, and vaccines. While we have not always been successful, we have learned over time how to save lives with public health and medical interventions that will ultimately see us to the other side of crises like COVID-19. Embracing "unprecedentedness" leaves us without the map our forebearers constructed through pain, struggle, ingenuity, and creativity, to survive our "Darwinian struggle" with disease (Snowden, 2020, p. 467; Snowden, 2021a). In short, we need a narrative framework rooted in precedence.

A RHETORIC OF PRECEDENCE AS *EQUIPMENT FOR LIVING* IN A PANDEMIC

Among the many consequences of the radical explosion in using the term "unprecedented" to classify (if not in any way clarify) our experiences during the pandemic is that we have failed to develop shared and robust resources for uniting the public to address it. In other words, we have lacked what the cultural and literary critic Kenneth Burke (1973) would have called "equipment for living" (p. 293) together during the pandemic. Burke (1973) emphasized the role of literature in generating such equipment, but we should not forget his goal was to promote a sort of "*sociological* criticism" (p. 293) offering insights that "apply beyond literature to life in general (thus helping to take literature out of its separate bin and give it a place in a general 'sociological' picture)" (p. 296). Burke also believed that all literature is implicated in the social, cultural, and political atmosphere of its time. It is not "pure" but rather a form of "medicine" (Burke, 1973, p. 293) that speaks to the pathologies of the moment. However, as a rhetorical scholar, Carly Woods (2009) noted, Burke's understanding of "medicine" implies the existence of both "good" and "bad" forms ("Medicine as Burke's Master Metaphor," para. 3). Indeed, in this sense, the rhetoric of *unprecedentedness is* a kind of equipment for dealing with the pandemic rooted in denial, ignorance, fear, and/or lack of attention to history.

As an alternative, I argue that the equipment we use to navigate this pandemic ought to be rooted in precedence. Indeed, as a form of Burkean medicine, precedence may act as a vaccination against unprecedentedness. As a kind of memory injection, precedence offers us resources to reveal the gaps in our historical narratives generated by claims of unprecedentedness. Here, I am offering an analogy to the way vaccines help our bodies develop memories of and defenses against disease. As the eminent immunologist Michael B. Oldstone (2020) noted in *Viruses, Plagues, & History: Past, Present, and Future*:

> *Immunologic memory* is the rapid and specific immune response programmed by a previous infection with that virus or immunization with its pharmaceutical counterpart. Thus, vaccines prime the immune system and program it to anticipate and resist future infection by the specific pathogens they represent. (pp. 304–305)[4]

As vaccines train our bodies to recognize and eliminate COVID-19, rhetorical and communication scholars committed to a rhetoric of precedence should craft narrative frameworks that bring our past into concordance with our present to discover a better future. When we move past the discordance of false unprecedentedness, we encounter a history filled with lessons about how to survive outbreaks.

Offering a particularly powerful example of the rhetoric of precedence, Snowden (2020) demonstrated how a variety of public health interventions had been developed across the centuries, some of which may be applicable to our time while others are not. Indeed, one of the keys to turning historical knowledge into actionable policy is careful attention to the differences that exist between the past and present. In a particularly important passage about the public health measures taken during outbreaks of the bubonic plague in past centuries, including "quarantine," Snowden (2020) argued:

> When new, virulent, and poorly understood epidemic diseases emerged, such as cholera and HIV/AIDS, the first reaction was to turn to the same defenses that

> appeared to have worked so effectively against plague. It was unfortunate that antiplague measures, however successfully deployed against bubonic plague, proved to be useless or even counterproductive when used against infections with profoundly different modes of transmission. In this manner, the plague regulations established a style of public health that remained a permanent temptation, partly because they were thought to have worked in the past and because, in a time of uncertainty and fear, they provided the reassuring sense of being able to do something. In addition, they conferred upon authorities the legitimating appearance of acting resolutely, knowledgeably, and in accord with precedent. (p. 81)

In order to effectively determine adequate "precedent" from the past, Snowden (2020) developed an eleven-part tool for comparative analysis of outbreaks that featured many questions related to causation, etiology, epidemiology, the natural course of the illness and case fatality rates, symptomology, victimology, transmission, virulence, and the like (pp. 83–87). We need to be equally rigorous as we consider just what historical narratives to pull forward into our experiences with COVID-19.

My approach to developing *equipment* relevant to our moment and capable of acting as an immunization against unprecedentedness involves discovering and applying the right precedents from our past. I argue that any effective, historically enriched, and narratively robust rhetorical immunization of this sort: (1) recognizes and actively advances ethical and useful historical analogies; (2) learns from efforts undertaken to address similar circumstances in the past (both effective and ineffective); and (3) acknowledges the wrongs committed in the past.[5] The first two of these criteria are evident in a brief case study presented in the next section on Taiwan's approach to addressing COVID-19 through the analogue of the earlier sudden acute respiratory syndrome (SARS) outbreak. The last is one that I take up in my conclusion, where I discuss the need to actively remember how health and justice have been undermined throughout the history of U.S. responses to emerging infectious diseases, pandemics, and healthcare in general.

LEARNING FROM THE PAST: THE "TAIWAN MODEL"

While the U.S. has faced many challenges implementing a national response to the COVID-19 pandemic, other nations have been at the forefront of developing strategies to contain and control the spread of this deadly disease. Taiwan has been at the forefront of these nations in large part because it has been highly effective at keeping infections down with a robust national response to the pandemic. The most crucial element of Taiwan's response was its grounding in an already well-developed public health infrastructure rooted in historical knowledge about the SARS outbreak it experienced in 2003. The case of Taiwan demonstrates not only that we need to frame pandemic outbreaks through historical understanding but also that constant attention to the lessons learned and careful efforts to implement them must work in tandem. It also shows how any effective approach to addressing pandemics requires careful attention to democratic culture and its rhetorical accoutrements, especially those related to legitimating public health initiatives that may limit freedom and autonomy to protect the common good.

In an article published in *Nature Immunology* in April 2021, Taiwan's Minister of Health and Welfare, Shih-Chung Chen (2021), outlined key tenets of the "Taiwan Model" (p. 393). Chen (2021) noted that as the outbreak emerged in Wuhan, many observers suggested Taiwan's "geographic proximity" (Chen, 2021, p. 393) to the origin of the pandemic in China would make it highly susceptible to severe rates of infection. But this did not occur. Why? Chen (2021) argued that Taiwan has been very effective in translating lessons learned from previous crises, especially the aforementioned SARS epidemic, into actual "reforms" (p. 393) to the health system and the cultivation of actionable knowledge in the present. Perhaps most important in this regard was Taiwan's creation of an institutional framework for dealing with disease outbreaks: the "Central Epidemic Command Center" (CECC) (Chen, 2021, p. 393), a part of its "National Health Command Center," which oversees several "disaster management" arenas from natural epidemics to bioterror attacks (Wang, Ng, & Brook, 2020, p. 1341). Thus, and despite its inability to participate in many international global health activities due to China's unwillingness to allow it into the WHO, Taiwan has been able to form and frame epidemic and pandemic policy more effectively than much of the rest of the world (Chen & Cohen, 2020).[6]

The foundation of Taiwan's strategy was the attention it paid to how SARS challenged its health infrastructure and made change necessary. Because it too is a coronavirus, SARS shares many similarities with COVID-19. As Snowden (2020) opined,

> [SARS] is a respiratory disease capable of spreading from person to person without a vector; it has an asymptomatic incubation period of more than a week; it generates symptoms that closely resemble those of other diseases; it takes a heavy toll on caregivers and hospital staff; it spreads easily and silently by air travel; and it has a CFR of 10%. (p. 471)

However, it is important to note that while it was more virulent (with a higher CFR or "case fatality rate") than COVID-19, its overall mortality was not as high. In other words, SARS was not as transmissible as COVID-19, so it did not go global in quite the same way. This was in part due to its "spread by droplets," which "requires extended contact for transmission, unlike classic airborne diseases such as influenza and smallpox" (Snowden, 2020, p. 473). Despite these differences, Chen (2021) pointed out that Taiwan noted key similarities and implemented an effective model to address COVID-19. In particular, Taiwan made use of "four major principles—rapid measures, early deployment, prudent actions, and transparency" (p.393). Chen (2021) emphasized, "We leveraged our democracy, the cooperation of citizens, and technology to overcome many challenges and created the 'Taiwan model' for combating the pandemic" (p. 393). Chen went on to unpack these principles, showing how at each stage of the pandemic, Taiwan responded to events as they unfolded with the use of quarantine measures, the development and distribution of supplies (e.g., masks), the ongoing review of current practices with an eye toward improvement, and the use of new communication technology to promote contact tracing and techniques to involve the broader community (including informative press conferences) in both understanding and acting against the pandemic (see also Wang, Ng, & Brook, 2020; Yeh & Cheng, 2020). In addition to these elements, Taiwan's "National Health Insurance" program, which "provid[es] universal coverage of healthcare services to all of citizens and residents legally residing in Taiwan" (Yeh & Cheng, 2020, p. 428), facilitated easy access to all services and materials necessary to track and treat the outbreak. Chen (2021) also pointed out how this national system allowed for easy collection and sharing of data about patients (p. 393).

At the end of this commentary, Chen (2021) argued: "COVID-19 has taught the world that it is important to always be prepared for an outbreak and to remain alert to any signs of an impending epidemic" (p. 393; see also Ding, 2014, p. 3). Indeed, but I would add, this is the one part of the document that failed to emphasize the deeper historical awareness upon which the "Taiwan Model" was developed. COVID-19 reaffirmed our need to be attentive; however, previous pandemics should have already taught this lesson. What is more, many of the insights gleaned from the 2003 SARS outbreak, especially quarantining, the use of masks, and related actions, have been part of public health methodology for centuries, starting with the bubonic plague and moving through other similar outbreaks with more or less successful results (Snowden 2020; 2021b).

Furthermore, the "Taiwan Model" was effective not only because it offered a variety of historically informed and, thus, evidence-based strategies for managing the biological spread of COVID-19. It also forestalled the emergence of a rhetorical pandemic of ignorance, fear, anxiety, and resistance from taking hold as it has in the U.S. Such reactions have been a common feature during past pandemics as well, not only when invasive measures were necessary to control the spread of illness but also when misunderstandings about pathogenesis, prevention, and cures were prevalent (Snowden, 2020). As such, the "Taiwan Model" is more than a public health approach to dealing with a pathogenic crisis. It is also a rhetorical approach to dealing with the threat of pathological communication and ideology that may emerge in pandemic life. As public health experts Ming-Jui Yeh and Yawen Cheng (2020), both of the Institute of Health Policy and Management at National Taiwan University in Taipei, have articulated, Taiwan's approach to addressing the rhetorical and ideological risks of pandemic life was rooted in effective leadership established through healthy democratic action. They pointed out that the CECC, noted previously, and Taiwan's Centers for Disease Control were afforded decision-making powers over state responses to pandemics in the aftermath of SARS. This control was established through legal means and as part of an informed deliberative process that continues, according to their account, to provide opportunities for engagement between government, corporations, and civil society.

Given this leadership architecture, Taiwan was able to overcome divisive elections and political divisions to approach the pandemic as a unified polity. As Yeh and Cheng (2020) noted, "With social cohesiveness, social trust, and citizen cooperation (after the competitive and seemingly splitting election), society quickly came together to fight the disease," an outcome they identified "as a legacy of democratization in Taiwan" (p. 432). What is more, they suggested that there are key aspects of Taiwanese political culture that have made the "Taiwan Model" effective including a more generalized social acceptance of masks as a typical hygienic tool. Finally, they argued that the geopolitical context of Taiwan has created a unique coincidence of democratic culture and internal unity against threats to the body politic: "particularly under China's external threats in the global arena, Taiwanese society has developed durable and resilient preparedness practices that can rapidly respond to any political and social challenges" (Yeh & Cheng, 2020, p. 432). In short, the "Taiwan Model" is ready to address the double pandemic. It has a health infrastructure informed by historical experience nestled within a democratic culture designed to facilitate a strong interface between government and civil society.

CONCLUSION: CULTIVATING RHETORICAL IMMUNITY AGAINST UNPRECEDENTEDNESS

As rhetorical theorist Kendall R. Phillips (2004) once noted, memory is "fluid and dynamic" and "open to contest, revision, and rejection" (p. 2). Phillips further stated: "To speak of memory in this way is to speak of a highly rhetorical process" (p. 2). Memory is not history, and history can be lost in the rhetorical reworking and even obliteration of memory over time (Phillips 2004; 2010). For example, in *Polio Wars: Sister Elizabeth Kenny and the Golden Age of American Medicine*, the historian of medicine Naomi Rogers (2014) demonstrated how a key historical figure in the development of physical therapy treatments for polio, Sister Elizabeth Kenny, was largely forgotten. This is due in large part to her nontraditional approach to medical practice and research, her gender (as a female, which in the 1940s and 1950s was often used to undermine and delegitimate her work), and the development of vaccinations which made treating polio less crucial than preventing it. Channeling similar ideas to those expressed by Phillips, Rogers (2014) noted at the end of the study that the history of public engagement (or lack thereof) with Kenny "illustrates the fragility of memory" and the nature of forgetting as an "active" endeavor (p. 425). We lose our past not only because it tends to erode over time through generational turnover and the frailty of our minds but also because we actively choose not to remember, especially when stories do not fit with our preconceptions, goals, and agendas.

Moreover, public memory cannot be cultivated in a vacuum. It is not merely about creating memorials, monuments, or textual artifacts. It is also about open dialogues and discussions about the past, a mode of engagement disallowed, or at least occluded, by rhetorics of unprecedentedness. As philosopher Edward S. Casey (2004) argued, public memory must be actively fostered "through ongoing interchange of ideas and thoughts, opinions and beliefs. It is just because public memory is so much in the arena of open discussion and debate that it is also subject to revision or, for that matter, resumption" (p. 30; see also Browne, 2004). Revising our understanding of the past and resuming its relevance in our lives requires piercing the boundaries between now and then through ongoing dialogue rooted in historical, experiential, and analogical narratives that are robust, inclusive, and just. The *discordant pandemic narratives* wrought over the past year and a half, many rooted in the rhetoric of unprecedentedness, have undermined both the formation of memory and its use in public dialogue. We must rediscover concordance between past and present in order to balance our minds and bodies with our new viral ecology.

The previous sections have articulated history as a rhetorical and pragmatic resource for addressing the challenges we may face during pandemic outbreaks. I have made a case for looking back to understand the present and construct a better future. I do not mean to suggest that what is happening now has happened in *exactly* the same way in our past. There are crucial differences in culture, politics, and economics. In the case of pandemics, there are also key distinctions in terms of not only disease etiology and epidemiology but also available technological and social interventions (Snowden, 2020). However, there are also valuable analogies that we must reengage. Rhetorical immunization against the discordances between not only our past and present but also our current biological realities and attitudes may, in part, be accomplished by seeking out narratives that demonstrate the power of historical knowledge in addressing contemporary problems. The case of Taiwan supplies just such an example as do larger historical narratives about epidemics and pandemics like those offered by Ding (2014), Oldstone (2020), Rogers (1992; 2014), and Snowden (2020; 2021a–c). These resources not only provide lessons to follow but also insights about previous failures in public health efforts.

We also need to recognize not only our previous public health failures but also those related to securing justice, the third element of my rhetoric of precedence as outlined earlier. As Snowden (2020) wrote, "The epidemic diseases that afflict a community are never purely random. They exploit features of a society that are social, economic, political, and environmental" (p. 234). Racism and other modes of oppression have been and continue to be determinative features of U.S. culture, impacting outcomes for individuals and communities across the political, socio-economic, and healthcare landscapes. They also cultivate distrust and hesitancy to accept new treatments and interventions. These factors have augmented the consequences of COVID-19 in the U.S., where BIPOC, LGBTQ+, and additional traditionally marginalized communities have suffered more complex and significant health and economic consequences (Andraska et al., 2021; Espina & Narruhn, 2021).

In sum, throughout this chapter, I have suggested that we are experiencing a double pandemic, one biological and the other rhetorical. To survive this double crisis, we need more than a vaccine for COVID-19. We need to invest in the recovery and ongoing dissemination of historical knowledge about previous pandemics that can supply us with equipment for survival. We need to embrace a rhetoric of precedence and its attendant curation and maintenance of public memory to counteract the discordances of the unprecedented circulating in pandemic life.

NOTES

1. Thank you to the editors, Sarina Chen, Joyce Chen, and Nicole Allaire, for their guidance and support during the writing of this chapter. Special thanks to Matthew P. Brigham (James Madison University) for reading drafts and providing invaluable feedback and Brendan Hughes (MSU Denver) for a timely reading recommendation.

2. I am not the first to use the language of a "double" or "dual" pandemic. Many in the media, public health, and medicine have used this language to emphasize related crises occurring in tandem with COVID-19, the most salient of which are systemic racism and its consequences for public health including ongoing and

significant disparities in health outcomes and inequitable access to health resources (see e.g., Espina & Narruhn, 2021). Others include, for example, the mental health consequences of the social and cultural changes wrought by the pandemic (see e.g., Pandey et al., 2021, p. 164). Moreover, the idea that biological epidemics may have associated rhetorical and cultural pathologies has been investigated previously, especially by Paula A. Treichler (1999) who focused on the "*epidemic of signification*" (p. 1) that encircled the HIV/AIDS epidemic in the U.S. Likewise, the technical and professional communication scholar Huiling Ding (2014) has studied "the construction of SARS as a social/cultural disease, in addition to being a medical one" (p. 23). Also of note is Naomi Rogers's (1992) recovery of discourses that associated "dirt and disease" (title and throughout) during early twentieth-century outbreaks of polio in the U.S. which tended to occlude more accurate understandings of the disease's etiology and epidemiology.

3. Please note that the numbers returned for these searches differ slightly from day to day. News aggregator databases like *Access World News—Historical and Current* may have access to different numbers of publications at different times depending on feeds, changes in content availability, and changes in agreements with content creators. Also, to keep the comparisons simple, I focused on one term for the pandemic: "COVID-19." Additional work to track "coronavirus," "SARS-CoV-2," "pandemic," etc., is planned for future iterations of this project. I also plan to track other uses of the term unprecedented in theses results that have little or nothing to do with the pandemic to see what other rhetorical insights may be gleaned from the circulation of this term.

4. I was inspired to make this move by rhetorical scholars Luke A. Winslow and Rebecca Lanier (2021), who have argued for the development of a "*rhetorical* herd immunity" (pp. 24–26, emphasis in original) in response to pathological rhetorics deployed by President Trump and his administration throughout the COVID-19 pandemic. I am also influenced here by work in social psychology to use a variety of argumentative "inoculation" strategies to ameliorate the rising influence of misinformation in public and political decision making (Lewandowsky & van der Linden, 2021).

5. Of course, there are risks associated with unethical and false historical analogies that drive misunderstanding and fear. Ding (2014) offered some examples of problematic analogies that emerged during the 2003 SARS epidemic, especially those rooted in "existing cultural biases about China" (p. 142; also see pp. 138–142, 177).

6. Despite its major successes, Taiwan did experience a spike in COVID-19 cases and deaths from May to August 2021 (Worldometer, 2021b). According to Yvette Tan (2021), writing for *BBC News*, experts have noted several potential causes, including focusing attention on controlling entry into the country as opposed to other strategies that would reduce the risk of outbreaks inside its borders.

REFERENCES

American Psychological Association. (2020). *Stress in America 2020: A national mental health crisis.* Retrieved from https://www.apa.org/news/press/releases/stress/2020/sia-mental-health-crisis.pdf

Andraska, E. A., Alabi, O., Dorsey, C., Erben, Y., Velazquez, G., Franco-Mesa, C., & Sachdev, U. (2021). Health care disparities during the COVID-19 pandemic. *Seminars in Vascular Surgery, 33*(4), 82–88. Retrieved from https://doi.org/10.1053/j.semvascsurg.2021.08.002

Aristotle. (1926a). *Art of rhetoric* (J. H. Freese, Trans.). Loeb Classical Library, Number 193. Cambridge, MA: Harvard University Press. (Original work published ca. 350 B.C.E.)

Aristotle. (1926b). *Nicomachean ethics* (H. Rackham, Trans.) Loeb Classical Library, Number 73. Cambridge, MA: Harvard University Press. (Original work published ca. 350 B.C.E.)

Browne, S. H. (2004). Arendt, Eichmann, and the politics of remembrance. In K. R. Phillips (Ed.), *Framing public memory* (pp. 45–64). Tuscaloosa: University of Alabama Press.

Burke, K. (1952). *A grammar of motives*. New York: Prentice-Hall, Inc.

Burke, K. (1966). Terministic screens. In K. Burke, *Language as symbolic action: Essays on life, literature, and method* (pp. 44–62). Berkeley: University of California Press.

Burke, K. (1973). Literature as equipment for living. In K. Burke, *The philosophy of literary form: Studies in symbolic action* (3rd ed.) (pp. 293–304). Berkeley: University of California Press.

Casey, E. S. (2004). Public memory in place and time. In K. R. Phillips (Ed.), *Framing public memory* (pp. 17–44). Tuscaloosa: University of Alabama Press.

Centers for Disease Control and Prevention (CDC). (2021, August 24). Vaccine safety given the speed of vaccine development and rollout (A section in *Answering patients' questions about COVID-19 vaccine and vaccination: Information for healthcare providers, pharmacists, and other vaccine providers*). *CDC*.gov. Retrieved from https://www.cdc.gov/vaccines/covid-19/hcp/answering-questions.html#vaccine-safety

Chen, S-C. (2021). Taiwan's experience in fighting COVID-19. *Nature Immunology, 22*, 393–394. Retrieved from https://doi.org/10.1038/s41590-021-00908-2

Chen, Y-J., & Cohen, J. A. (2020, April 9). Why does the WHO exclude Taiwan? *Council on Foreign Relations*. Retrieved from https://www.cfr.org/in-brief/why-does-who-exclude-taiwan

Ding, H. (2014). *Rhetoric of a global epidemic: Transcultural communication about SARS*. Carbondale: Southern Illinois University Press.

Epstein, S. (1995). The construction of lay expertise: AIDS activism and the forging of credibility in the reform of clinical trials. *Science, Technology, & Human Values, 20*(4), 408–437. Retrieved from https://doi.org/10.1177/016224399502000402

Espina, C. R., & Narruhn, R. A. (2021). "I can't breathe": Biopower in the time of COVID-19: An exploration of how biopower manifests in the dual pandemics of

COVID and racism. *Advances in Nursing Science*, *44*(3), 183–194. Retrieved from https://doi.org/10.1097/ANS.0000000000000355

France, D. (2012). *How to survive a plague*. [Film]. Public Square Films and Ninety Thousand Words.

Global Preparedness Monitoring Board (GPMB). (2019). *A world at risk: Annual report on global preparedness for health emergencies*. World Health Organization. Retrieved from https://www.gpmb.org/annual-reports/overview/item/2019-a-world-at-risk

Global Preparedness Monitoring Board. (2020). *A world in disorder: Global Preparedness Monitoring Board annual report 2020*. World Health Organization. Retrieved from https://www.gpmb.org/annual-reports/overview/item/2020-a-world-in-disorder

Global Preparedness Monitoring Board. (2021). *A world prepared: Global Preparedness Monitoring Board strategic plan 2021–2023*. Retrieved from https://www.gpmb.org/annual-reports/overview/item/gpmb-strat-plan-2021-2023

Google Trends. (n.d.). Unprecedented. Retrieved from https://trends.google.com/trends/explore?date=all&geo=US&q=unprecedented

Harper, K. (2017). *The fate of Rome: Climate, disease, and the end of an empire*. Princeton, NJ: Princeton University Press.

Holden, S. (2012, September 20). They wouldn't take no for an answer in the battle against AIDS. *New York Times*. Retrieved from https://www.nytimes.com/2012/09/21/movies/how-to-survive-a-plague-aids-documentary-by-david-france.html

Knodel, J. (2020, March 24). Texas Lt. Gov. Dan Patrick suggests he, other seniors willing to die to get economy going again. *NBC News*. Retrieved from https://www.nbcnews.com/news/us-news/texas-lt-gov-dan-patrick-suggests-he-other-seniors-willing-n1167341

Lewandowsky, S., & van der Linden, S. (2021). Countering misinformation and fake news through inoculation and prebunking. *European Review of Social Psychology*, *32*(2), 348–384. Retrieved from http://doi.org/10.1080/10463283.2021.1876983

Lin, C. A. (2020). A year like no other: A call to curb the infodemic and depoliticize a pandemic crisis. *Journal of Broadcasting & Electronic Media*, *64*(5), 661–671. Retrieved from https://doi.org/10.1080/08838151.2020.1871185

McGee, M. C. (1990). Text, context, and the fragmentation of contemporary culture. *Western Journal of Speech Communication*, *54*(3), 274–289. Retrieved from https://doi.org/10.1080/10570319009374343

Mitchell, G. R., & McTigue, K. M. (2007). The U.S. obesity "epidemic": Metaphor, method, or madness? *Social Epistemology*, *21*(4), 391–423. Retrieved from https://doi.org/10.1080/02691720701746557

Oldstone, M. B. A. (2020). *Viruses, plagues, & history: Past, present, and future*. New York: Oxford University Press.

Oxford English Dictionary (OED). (2021a, June). Precedent, noun. *OED Online*. Oxford University Press. Retrieved from https://www-oed-com.aurarialibrary.idm.oclc.org/view/Entry/149572?rskey=Jyvfh7&result=1&isAdvanced=false#eid

Oxford English Dictionary. (2021b, June). Unprecedented, adj. *OED Online*. Oxford University Press. Retrieved from https://www-oed-com.aurarialibrary.idm.oclc.org/view/Entry/216439?redirectedFrom=unprecedented&

Palmer, K. (2021a, August 25). Barrier removed (A section in *Debt relief now could help PCC in long run—Millions in student loans are forgiven by college's board*). *The Arizona Daily Star*, A001.

Palmer, K. (2021b, August 25, updated November 24). As PCC's enrollment lags, forgiving $2.7M of student debt may offer boost. *The Arizona Daily Star*. Retrieved from https://tucson.com/news/local/subscriber/as-pccs-enrollment-lags-forgiving-2-7m-of-student-debt-may-offer-boost/article_177119cc-0468-11ec-a6ac-9f51d8e86eae.html

Pandey, K., Thurman, M., Johnson, S. D., Acharya, A., Johnston, M., Klug, E. A., Olwenyi, O. A., Rajaiah, R., & Byrareddy, S. N. (2021). Mental health issues during and after COVID-19 vaccine era. *Brain Research Bulletin, 176*, 161–173. Retrieved from https://doi.org/10.1016/j.brainresbull.2021.08.012

Park, A. (2021a, July 28). Simone Biles' Olympic team final withdrawal could help athletes put their mental health first. *Time*. Retrieved from https://time.com/6084499/simone-biles-mental-health-olympics/

Park, A. (2021b, August 8). How the Tokyo Olympics changed the conversation about athletes' mental health. *Time*. Retrieved from https://time.com/6088078/mental-health-olympics-simone-biles/

Pezenik, S. (2021, August 23). FDA grants full approval to Pfizer COVID-19 vaccine. *ABC News*. Retrieved from https://abcnews.go.com/Politics/fda-grants-full-approval-pfizer-covid-19vaccine/story?id=79599488

Phillips, K. R. (2004). Introduction. In K. R. Phillips (Ed.), *Framing public memory* (pp. 1–14). Tuscaloosa: University of Alabama Press.

Phillips, K. R. (2010). The failure of memory: Reflections on rhetoric and public remembrance. *Western Journal of Communication, 74*(2), 208–223. Retrieved from https://doi.org/10.1080/10570311003680600

Preston, R. (2020). *Crisis in the red zone: The story of the deadliest Ebola outbreak in history, and of the viruses to come*. New York: Random House.

Rogers, N. (1992). *Dirt and disease: Polio before FDR.* New Brunswick, NJ: Rutgers University Press.

Rogers, N. (2014). *Polio wars: Sister Elizabeth Kenny and the golden age of American medicine.* New York: Oxford University Press.

Snowden, F. M. (2020). *Epidemics and society: From the Black Death to the present* (New Preface). New Haven, CT: Yale University Press.

Snowden, F. M. (2021a). Lecture 10—Asiatic cholera (II): Five pandemics. *Epidemics in western society since 1600.* [Audiovisual recording]. Open Yale Courses. (Lecture originally given in spring 2010). Retrieved from https://oyc.yale.edu/history/hist-234/lecture-10

Snowden, F. M. (2021b). Lecture 20—Pandemic influenza. *Epidemics in western society since 1600.* [Audiovisual recording]. Open Yale Courses. (Lecture originally given in spring 2010). Retrieved from https://oyc.yale.edu/history/hist-234/lecture-20

Snowden, F. M. (2021c). Lecture 25—SARS, avian influenza, and swine flu: Lessons and prospects. *Epidemics in western society since 1600.* [Audiovisual recording]. Open Yale Courses. (Lecture originally given in spring 2010). Retrieved from https://oyc.yale.edu/history/hist-234/lecture-25.

Splete, H. (2021, August 6). Fauci says "unprecedented" conditions could influence COVID vaccine approval for kids. *The Hospitalist.* Retrieved from https://www.the-hospitalist.org/hospitalist/article/244007/pediatrics/fauci-says-unprecedented-conditions-could-influence-covid

Tan, Y. (2021, May 20). COVID-19: What went wrong in Singapore and Taiwan? *BBC News*. Retrieved from https://www.bbc.com/news/world-asia-57153195

Treichler, P. A. (1999). *How to have theory in an epidemic: Cultural chronicles of AIDS*. Durham, NC: Duke University Press.

Trump, D. J. (2020, March 11). Read President Trump's speech on coronavirus: Full transcript. [Speech Transcript]. *New York Times*. Retrieved from https://www.nytimes.com/2020/03/11/us/politics/trump-coronavirus-speech.html

Wang, C. J., Ng, C. Y., & Brook, R. H. (2020). Response to COVID-19 in Taiwan: Big data analytics, new technology, and proactive testing. *Journal of the American Medical Association*, *323*(14), 1341–1342. Retrieved from https://doi.org/10.1001/jama.2020.3151

Winslow, L. A., & Lanier, R. A. (2021, November 20). Thinning the herd: COVID-19, immunity, and the rhetoric of Trumpian catastrophe. [Conference paper]. National Communication Association's 107th Annual Convention. Seattle, Washington.

Woods, C. (2009). "Everything is medicine": Burke's master metaphor? *KB Journal: The Journal of the Kenneth Burke Society*, *5*(2). Retrieved from https://www.kbjournal.org/carly_woods

Worldometer. (2021a, November 28). COVID-19 coronavirus pandemic. Retrieved from https://www.worldometers.info/coronavirus/

Worldometer. (2021b, September 22). Taiwan. Retrieved from https://www.worldometers.info/coronavirus/country/taiwan/

Yeh, M-J., & Cheng, Y. (2020, November 6). Policies tackling the COVID-19 pandemic: A sociopolitical perspective from Taiwan. *Health Security*, *18*(6), 427–434. Retrieved from https://doi.org/10.1089/hs.2020.0095

Zimmer, K. (2021, August 9). Dissecting the unusual biology of the SARS-CoV-2 Delta Variant. *The Scientist: Exploring Life, Inspiring Innovation*. Retrieved from https://www.the-scientist.com/newsopinion/dissecting-the-unusual-biology-of-the-sars-cov-2-delta-variant-69068

Chapter Six

Discordant Rhetorical Responses

Crisis Communication in Sports Organizations in the COVID-19 Pandemic

Tyler Welsh, R. Tyler Spradley,
and Elizabeth Spradley

Former Ebola Czar Ron Klain argues that the most crucial factor in combating a viral pandemic is "mustering all of government effectively, efficiently and quickly to fight [the] disease" (Debenedetti, 2020, para. 2). Nigerian physician Dr. Adaora Okoli, reflecting on lessons learned while fighting the Ebola breakout in her home country, states, "Viruses don't wait for governments to act. You can have all the resources, the money, the people, but if you don't act fast, the virus will outpace you" (Holeyman, 2020, para. 31). These public health officials both highlight the urgency of a rapid response to a viral pandemic. That same urgency is present in the fight against the most recent pandemic, COVID-19. World Health Organization Director Tedros Adhanom Ghebreyesus recently praised several countries for their swift, dramatic response to the COVID-19 outbreak. He specifically singled out New Zealand, a country that started taking preventative measures a mere three days after the WHO declared the outbreak a public health emergency (Partridge-Hicks, 2020). However, as COVID-19 began to spread across the United States in early 2020, it became clear that leadership and public health authorities did not have a unified message. The federal response labored slowly, ultimately deferring to state and local authorities. The effect of this chaotic, slow response is undeniable: the United States now has confirmed nearly thirty-six million cases, and almost 615,778 people have died at the time of writing (CDC, 2021).

The failed US government response is one of many examples of leadership responding slowly and inadequately to the coronavirus pandemic. The world of professional sports also provides case studies of organizations and their leaders attempting to adapt to the COVID-19 pandemic. Two leagues in particular—the National Football League (NFL) and the National Basketball Association (NBA)—provide examples of how organizations have attempted to handle the disease safely while remaining operational. The disparate responses from these two organizations raise a centralizing question: How did two of America's largest national sports leagues negotiate discordant rhetoric, guidelines, and laws to achieve pandemic iterations of "open for business"? The NBA decided to immediately suspend their season, and it was not until the league was able to construct a quarantined "bubble" that it allowed games to begin again. On the other hand, the NFL had over six months to strategize and implement a functional protocol in response to Covid-19. While it established league-wide guidelines, the NFL ultimately delegated many decisions to individual franchises. This chapter examines the results and implications of these discordant responses.

The cultural arena of sports offers a unique lens through which to view human behavior and communication. Leadership within sports teams and organizations is a vital component of success both on and off the field. Leaders in influential organizations such as the NBA and the NFL often feel extreme pressure to provide information, but lack experience with such large-scale crises like a pandemic, and such inexperience can lead to defensive rhetoric and poor decision-making. This chapter examines how leaders within sports organizations might strategize their communication styles to offer better paths for acting effectively, efficiently, and quickly to fight crises like global pandemics in the future. To do so, this chapter, "Discordant Rhetorical Responses: Crisis Communication in Sports Organizations in the COVID-19 Pandemic" is structured as follows. To begin, a review of sport crisis communication scholarship clarifies what is meant by sport and crisis communication as they intersect and come to bear on the study of sport crisis leadership. Then, the chapter offers a qualitative thematic analysis of the NBA and NFL commissioners' rhetorical responses to the coronavirus pandemic as a way to study sport crisis leadership. In examining direct rhetoric from the NBA's commissioner Adam Silver and the NFL's commissioner Roger Goodell, discordant themes emerge from their respective sport crisis leadership. Finally, this chapter draws on the discordant rhetoric and leadership literature to suggest best practices to guide sports organizations and their leaders to more effectively communicate in crises.

SPORT CRISIS COMMUNICATION LITERATURE

Sports organizations and their stakeholders are not immune from crisis events disrupting operations. Athletes and sports organizations experience reputational crises from a myriad of accusations of wrongdoing in their personal and professional endeavors (e.g., Blaney, Lippert, & Smith, 2013). Sports arenas are subject to security threats ranging from terrorism (e.g., Spaaij, 2016) to anti-social—even violent—fan behavior (e.g., Newson, 2019). Natural disasters and pandemics disrupt community, collegiate, and professional leagues' seasons and individual sporting events (e.g., DiFiori et al., 2021; Wicker et al., 2013). The list of sport crises is long and wide, spurring a dearth of scholarship at the intersection of communication, crisis, and sports. The literature on sport crisis communication, while limited, examines the varied responses of sports organizations, athletes, media, and fans to crisis (Harker & Saffer, 2018). Positioned as a subfield intersecting with "communication, mass communication, public relations, sport communication, and crisis communication" (Harker & Saffer, 2018, p. 370), sport crisis communication examines anticipatory (e.g., crisis planning, risk communication) and reactionary (e.g., image repair, policy changes) approaches to the crisis. To better understand what *is* and *is not* sport crisis communication, this chapter draws on the following frameworks and definitions, culminating in a concise definition from which the chapter proceeds.

Breaking down the term *sport crisis communication*, the definitions for sport communication and crisis communication come into focus. First, sport communication encompasses mediated and face-to-face interactions across various levels of communication (e.g., interpersonal, group, organizational, public, and mass media) in the context of sports. Scholarly attention to sport communication within the field of communication has led to interest groups and divisions in the major communication associations in the US and internationally as well as an international organization dedicated to communication and sport (Ishak, 2017), and the *Routledge Handbook of Sport Communication* was published in 2013 as further evidence of the fast-paced growth of sport communication as an established sub-field in communication (Pedersen, 2013). This chapter draws on the aforementioned definition and the body of work in sport communication as it intersects with crisis communication.

Second, crisis communication is catalyzed by a crisis, a triggering event of natural or man-made causes (Spradley, 2017). Despite the ubiquity of crises in the present, crises pose unique challenges for organizations and their leaders. Hermann's (1963) description of crisis events and their impact on organizations is summative. Hermann (1963) argues that crises are surprising events that exceed organizational expectations, threaten the standard means of organizational operation, and require a swift, effective response. Seeger and Sellnow (2016) clarify the definition of crisis communication "as the ongoing process of creating shared meaning among and between groups, communities, individuals, and agencies, within the ecological context of a crisis, for the purpose of preparing for and reducing, limiting, and responding to threats and harms" (p. 13). Crisis communication scholars are interested in concurrently understanding and prescribing the role of communication in crisis events to prevent, mitigate, and recover (Spradley, 2017). Considering definitional clarity given to both sport and crisis communication, we offer a working definition for sport crisis communication. Sport crisis communication is the meaning-making process to anticipate, respond, and recover from crisis events in sport contexts.

One particularly vibrant strand of research in sport crisis communication focuses on image. Crises threaten reputations or images, and image threats can constitute a crisis (Coombs & Holladay, 2008). Harker and Saffer's (2018) twenty-five-year meta-analysis of sport crisis communication research identifies image repair theory (IRT) as the most prolific theoretical perspective within the sport crisis communication subfield. Advanced in large part by the work of William Benoit (1995), IRT has been used to study athletes' responses to accusations of wrongdoing, including auto racer Tony Stewart (Jerome, 2008), basketball player Kobe Bryant (Meng & Pan, 2013), the Duke lacrosse team (Fortunato, 2008), football player Ben Roethlisberger (Meng & Pan, 2013), football player Terrell Owens (Brazeal, 2008), golfer Tiger Woods (Farhi, 2010; Meng & Pan, 2013), figure skater Tonya Harding (Benoit & Hanczor, 1994), swimmer Michael Phelps (Walsh & McAllister-Spooner, 2011), and many more (see the edited volume by Blaney et al., 2013). Yet another strand of sport crisis communication research focused on reputation uses another popular theoretical framework from crisis communication—Situational Crisis Communication Theory (SCCT) (Coombs, 2018). For example, Jackson and Thaker (2021) examine New Zealand's renowned rugby player Aaron Smith's image-threatening controversy nicknamed *toilet tryst*. In their analysis, SCCT's framework enables comparison between the messaging of Smith, his management, the rugby team, media, and fans. Similarly, Brown and associates (2015) drew on SCCT in their examination of Penn State's and sport fans' communication in response to the firing of football coach Joe Paterno, and his proximity to the Sandusky child molestation scandal. In each of these examples, fans' social media messaging functioned to repair or defend the tarnished images in question, which underscores the need to examine a variety of stakeholder communication in relation to sport crisis image repair rhetoric.

As sport crisis communication continues to expand, we seek to add another strand of research—*sport crisis leadership communication.* In other words, we seek to understand the intersections of communication, crisis, and leadership in sport contexts. Arguably, much of the research on sport crisis communication has implications for sport crisis leadership communication practices. For example, the work in IRT suggests that sport leaders accused of wrongdoing benefit from corrective action and mortification communication strategies (see Brazeal, 2008). Therefore, we turn to the focus of this chapter—discordant rhetorical responses between the NFL and the NBA leadership, specifically the themes that emerge from the rhetoric of their commissioners. This study further whittles down the focus in sport crisis communication to leadership within sport crisis communication.

THEMATIC ANALYSIS OF SPORT CRISIS LEADERSHIP IN COVID-19

In the wake of the emergent COVID-19 virus, all industries were tasked with making difficult decisions in order to adapt to the volatile conditions imposed on the world. Sports organizations were no exception. All major professional sports leagues struggled to implement new health policies that would protect not only their teams and players, but also their spectators. The rhetoric that emerged from leaders in sports organizations communicated *sport crisis leadership* through their rhetorical acts. This chapter explores two professional sport leaders' rhetorical responses to COVID-19 in 2020—the NBA's Adam Silver and the NFL's Roger Goodell. Collecting sports media articles with direct communication from Silver and Goodell, this rhetorical analysis follows Zompetti's (2019) lead by identifying themes in the commissioners' communication that constituted their rhetorical approaches to sport crisis leadership. This section reviews the data set and analytic method used.

Data Collection

In order to reveal the emergent themes within each individual's sports crisis leadership, we sought to gather direct communication from each league leader. Both leaders utilized the medium of league-wide memos to communicate to teams and franchises how to respond to the ensuing public health crisis. For Silver, we looked at several (N = 8) mainstream press articles that quoted directly from league-wide memos written by him and include direct quotes from public statements he made in press conferences and interviews. These articles were selected because they offer the clearest examples of Silver's communication style and word choices. Additionally, the articles detailing the memos cover an important span of time (March 2020 to August 2020) when the COVID-19 pandemic began to spread. These articles were published on sports media websites such as NBA.com and ESPN.com and were found through keyword searches on mainstream search engines.

Similarly, to analyze Goodell's pandemic response, we looked at eight (N = 8) leaguewide memos written by Goodell and distributed to all NFL teams. These memos were initially private but made public by various sports media journalists on the social media platform Twitter. These documents were obtained by keyword searches within Twitter's advanced archive search. We argue that these direct memos are the most succinct way to examine Goodell's sport crisis leadership because they are his exact words communicated to teams within the league. While this dataset does not fully encompass each leader's response entirely, they offer instructions, warnings, protocols, and rhetoric that seeks to directly respond to the conditions of the ensuing pandemic. In limiting our dataset to direct league memos and public statements, we argue these artifacts sufficiently represent the direct communication of each individual's crisis leadership rhetoric.

Data Analysis: Thematic Analysis

Thematic analysis is a prominent approach to analyzing rhetorical data. Rhetorical scholars have applied thematic approaches to study a diversity of rhetorical exigencies like instructional intercultural rhetoric (Delante, 2020), political communication on social media (Zompetti, 2019), the rhetoric of movements (Sedano, 1980). This study employs thematic analysis to study the rhetorical exigency surrounding the need for sport crisis leaders to respond to the coronavirus pandemic in 2020. The basic process of thematic analysis is a close read of the data to attend to categories, patterns, and repetitions in the language (Braun & Clarke, 2012; Zompetti, 2019). More specifically, we looked to the specific steps of thematic analysis laid out by interpretive scholars Braun and Clarke (2006; 2012), which differentiate thematic analysis from other inductive methods such as grounded theory (Braun & Clarke, 2019). Inductive reasoning is applied to data through a flexible coding process outlined in the following steps: time spent with data, initial and flexible coding of data, thematic coding of data, review of the theme, clarification of themes (e.g., labels, definitions, criteria), and writing (Braun & Clarke, 2006). Themes are not "in the data" but are, instead, generated by the researcher from the language, categories, and repetitions noted within the data (Braun & Clarke, 2019, p. 593). For Braun and Clark, themes are central organizing concepts constituted by their "shared meaning *underpinned* or united by a core concept" (p. 593, emphasis in the original).

We applied the step-by-step thematic analysis as follows. For the sake of coherency, the first author led the data collection, data review, and initial coding, and the second and third authors stepped in to discuss initial coding and finalize themes, clarify themes, and write. We argue that the comparative thematic analysis of Silver's and Goodell's sport crisis leadership demonstrates differing responses, which culminate in *discordant* sport crisis leadership.

Furthermore, we assert that Silver's rhetoric reflects the dominant rhetorical approach to sport crisis communication, subsequently driving the NBA toward a decisive and quick solution to the situation. Conversely, we examine Goodell's rhetoric as a discordant rhetorical approach to sport crisis communication that deviates and deflects from taking decisive action in a pandemic crisis.

SILVER'S SPORT CRISIS LEADERSHIP

The outbreak of COVID-19 emerged while the NBA was in the middle of its 2019–2020 season and was the first of America's four major professional sports to respond to the pandemic. Silver's utilization of sport crisis leadership was instrumental in setting the parameters and expectations for how leaders should act and communicate when faced with a public health emergency. We examine three themes and the narratives that emerge from Silver's response: (1) centralization of response, (2) emphasis on caution, and (3) decisive (top-level) action. These three emergent themes comprise the rhetoric of Silver's sport crisis leadership, and we argue they offer a dominant response in the wake of the COVID-19 outbreak.

Centralization of Response

When a crisis hits an organization, members should know unequivocally where to look and listen for directions. Silver's response to the virus communicated clear recommendations, restrictions, and updates for teams to adhere to. Journalist Tim Reynolds (2020b, para. 2) notes that as early as March 2nd, the commissioner's office released memos to all teams offering "10 recommendations to players with hopes of decreasing risks of getting the virus." These suggestions included avoiding high fives with fans, not signing autographs, and other standard precautions for illness prevention. Additionally, the memo explained the commissioner's office was working in tandem with "infectious disease experts, including the Centers for Disease Control and infectious disease researchers at Columbia University in New York" (Reynolds, 2020b, para. 3). This language established an early tone in the response, informing the league that guidelines would be channeled through the commissioner's office and distributed directly to teams. Additionally, the memo created a hierarchy with Silver positioned on top of the centralized response but also notes that he is open to collaboration with the NBA Players Association, leading experts, and team physicians. This centralized response theme coheres to a dominant sports crisis leadership response because it reduces ambiguity regarding direction and instructions. While there is communication that reflects collaboration in the decision-making process, Silver's sport crisis leadership indicates that the response derives unilaterally from his office.

Silver's centralized response continued to grow and adapt as testing for the virus became available. With few tests available, NBA players started to be monitored at a frequency most common citizens could not access. Some critics alluded to this access as preferential treatment, with New York City mayor Bill de Blasio tweeting, "with all due respect, an entire NBA team should NOT get tested for Covid-19 while there are critically ill patients waiting to be tested. Tests should not be for the wealthy, but for the sick" (de Blasio, 2020). De Blasio's critique was warranted as tests were difficult to acquire, and many patients were facing life-threatening scenarios. Silver responded to this criticism in an interview with CBS Sports stating,

> In the case of the NBA, we've been following the recommendations of public health officials . . . I understand from a public health standpoint why some people have reacted the way they did, but I'd say from an NBA standpoint we were following directives. (Herbert, 2020, para. 24)

This response establishes the narrative that while the NBA would work in conjunction with experts, ultimately, the league decisions and protocols came from Silver's office. Again, this crystallizes the theme of Silver's centralized response—teams would not be making their own individual decisions, and players would not be making their own protocols. Later memos would also require that players not engage in any non-essential travel and prohibited international travel, even for players who had citizenship abroad (Reynolds, 2020a). These directives were in concert with the closing of all team facilities (including both practice and training buildings) once players started testing positive. Repeatedly Silver's communication via memos and interviews reiterated that teams, players, and staff were to listen to his office in terms of guidance through the ever-shifting conditions of the crisis.

Emphasis on Caution

At the beginning of the pandemic, health and safety protocols were often advocating for an ad hoc approach to preventing transmission of the novel virus. Public health experts urged that no health protocol could be *too safe* given the many unknowns at the time. However, Silver established a theme of emphasizing caution well before any established professional sports league started implementing or drawing up safety guidelines. The NBA has offices located across the world, including several across the country of China. In January of 2020, Silver maintained close contact with staff and employees monitoring how the virus was spreading and wreaking havoc across the country in cities like Shanghai, Beijing, Hong Kong, and Taipei. In an interview with Rachel Nichols, Silver explained how this early caution started well before it became apparent the virus had reached the US, stating, "We've been living this at the league office since mid-January. We've been on alert as at least to what the consequences could be if the coronavirus had spread to the United States" (Shelburne, 2020, para. 19). In addition to the public interview, the commissioner's office released several memos, almost daily, urging caution and to prepare for new protocols.

This proactive communication evoked a norm of intense carefulness at a time when much of the public was unaware of what the growing crisis would entail. For years, Silver had kept David Weiss, an infectious disease liaison, on staff (Senior Vice President, Player Matters) at the NBA precisely for these types of crises. At the instruction of Silver, Weiss crafted daily memos as news of the growing virus spread. In a press conference on February 15th, Silver commented on the severity of the unfolding health crisis, "It's almost hard for us to be having conversations about the broadcasting of games when there's a major national, if not global, health crisis happening" (Shelburne, 2020, para. 22). This press conference was followed by several more memos urging caution and communication with local health officials. This rhetoric centered around the theme of risk aversion in which it underscored the severity of the impending spread of the virus, and it was constantly and quickly being communicated to all levels of the organization.

Another example of Silver's emphasis on caution was the choice to eliminate spectators from the stadiums in which games were played. In early March, the NBA, the NHL, and many professional sports leagues in Europe were still hosting games filled with tens of thousands of fans. Silver's inclination to remove fans from the stands was not a spur-of-the-moment decision. Instead, he began laying the groundwork as early as March 7th. In a memo released to all NBA teams, Silver informed teams they should be prepared to play "with only essential staff present" (Mahoney, 2020, para. 2). The idea of competitive sports without people in the seats cheering and screaming in support of their team was unimaginable. Yet, Silver remained steadfast in his communication that incoming data suggested large public gatherings could become "super spreader" events.

Silver's emphasis on caution did not go uncontested. Lebron James, perhaps the most publicly well-known current NBA player, voiced extreme dissent at the prospect of playing in empty stadiums, stating:

> We play games without the fans? Nah, that's impossible. I ain't playing if I ain't got the fans in the crowd. That's who I play for. I play for my teammates, and I play for the fans. . . . So if I show up to an arena and there ain't no fans in there, I ain't playing. They can do what they want to do. (Mahoney, 2020, para. 4)

The "they" in James's final sentence was a direct callout to Silver and a challenge of his authority. Despite the pushback, Silver's preference for caution continued to dominate the themes within his sport crisis leadership response. At the instruction of Silver, Vice President Weiss continued to send out daily memos emphasizing the need for teams to be prepared to coordinate with local medical officials. Furthermore, Silver's memos warned of the potentiality of "temperature checks on players, team staff, referees, and anyone else who is essential to conducting such a game in the team's arena" (Mahoney, 2020, para. 6). At every turn, Silver's rhetoric through memos and interviews communicated an expectation to reduce, mitigate, and eliminate health risks where possible. A centralized response and emphasis on caution clearly were themes that emerged from the web of discourse communicated by Silver.

These themes provided his organization with a clear chain of command and the notion to be as careful as possible.

Decisive Action

The novel nature of COVID-19 forced all citizens to be vigilant as new information and data were released regarding how the virus spread and the symptoms patients faced. Given the constant stream of daily information, decisions within organizations needed to constantly adapt and be open to change at a moment's notice. But beyond flexibility, leadership within organizations also needed to communicate *decisiveness* in order to retain hierarchies and establish new norms in the face of mounting challenges.

On March 11th, an Oklahoma City Thunder medical staffer ran up to game officials right before tip-off to inform the referees that a player had tested positive for COVID-19. This was the first publicly known positive case for the then new virus and Silver had only a few minutes to decide how to proceed. Silver reached out to the Oklahoma City health commissioner to see if they would mandate the shutdown of the game but received no response. In an interview with *USA Today*, Silver recounted the call he made: "I realized we had to err on the side of caution. There wasn't time to have a board meeting so I made a decision that we had to call that game" (Zillgitt & Medina,

2021, para. 41). Within minutes, fans were asked to leave the stands and go home as games across the league were postponed. An hour later, Silver released a public statement: "The NBA is suspending game play following the conclusion of tonight's schedule of games until further notice. The NBA will use this hiatus to determine next steps for moving forward in regard to the coronavirus pandemic" (Zillgitt & Medina, 2021, para. 51).

This moment was a critical turning point for not only sports, but the pandemic response in the country as a whole. Up until that halted game, recorded positive cases within the United States were rare. Silver's decisive choice to halt all league activity was instrumental in all professional sports leagues reassessing how they would respond to the growing threat of the virus. Silver's call to shut down the NBA quickly made the pandemic a reality, no longer a hypothetical. Dallas Mavericks owner Mark Cuban explained how Silver's decisive actions that day shifted his perspective on the situation:

> I was stunned . . . it immediately clarified that this was no longer about basketball, it was about the health and safety of our families and I had a lot to learn and think about in order to be able to take care of my family's health and to protect and help our friends and employees. (Zillgitt & Medina, 2021, para. 56)

Decisive actions and choices from leadership positions can communicate urgency and importance to audiences. Silver's fast response to the first positive test set a tone for how the NBA would decidedly work and communicate within the context.

Silver's next choice was perhaps the most decisive act of his sport crisis leadership—the decision to resume league play in a quarantined "bubble." On June 15th, over three months after the first positive player test, Silver delivered a one hundred-plus page document to league owners and players outlining the specifics of how the NBA would proceed to quarantine, test, and ultimately finish the 2019–2020 season (Bontemps, 2020). The document was thorough, outlining hundreds of protocol possible guidelines in order to best protect all the staff, players, and officials within the bubble. While other leagues such as Major League Baseball briefly considered the idea of a similar bubble, Silver was insistent on resuming play as quickly and safely as possible, explaining in a press conference that while "we can't outrun the virus," the bubble was "a closed network" (Aschburner, 2020, para. 3). Silver's decisive action for creating the bubble featured detailed planning and overly exhaustive rules and procedures. But it communicated with clarity to owners and players that this was not an ill-conceived plan. This paved the way for unanimous support within the league to proceed. Silver declared, "We believe we've developed a safe and responsible plan to restart the season" (Aschburner, 2020, para. 29).

The results of the decisive action were unequivocally clear. Zero positive test cases were returned during the entire quarantined period within the bubble (Oxner, 2020). And while the health and safety precautions proved to work demonstrably well, the decisive choice to construct and carry out the season in the bubble preserved $1.5 billion in revenue for the league (Lombardo, 2020). Yet, like most industries during the pandemic, the league still suffered serious financial shortages, and players commented on the toll the isolation of the bubble had on their mental health. But Silver's decisive action ensured players to safely and effectively finish the season, mitigating their potential financial loss. We identify that his sport crisis leadership offered a centralized, cautious, and decisive response to a challenging pandemic context. We argue that this response became a dominant one that provided a template for how sports organizations could respond in the future.

GOODELL'S SPORT CRISIS LEADERSHIP

Unlike the NBA, Roger Goodell had nearly six months to respond to and prepare for a season under pandemic conditions. In examining Goodell's communication, we argue he offers a *discordant* response to the dominant response established by Silver. What follows is a thematic analysis of Goodell's sport crisis leadership rhetoric. These themes include decentralized responses, adjustable risks, and indecisive reactions.

Decentralized Responses

The NFL closed its main offices on March 13th and directed club facilities to close on March 26th (ProFootballTalk, 2020). On April 6th, Goodell (2020a, posted in Pelissero's tweet, 2020a) wrote a memorandum to all teams informing them of the indefinite status of the closings and urged them to prepare for significant changes in the upcoming season. This communication was the first iteration of Goodell's sport crisis leadership, and while it, on the one hand, sought to establish a centralized response to the pandemic concerns, it also opened the door for a theme we identify as a more *decentralized* approach. The memo highlights each club's immense challenges in preparing for the draft but urges them to "comply with government directives and to model safe health practices" (Goodell, 2020a, p. 2, posted in Pelissero, 2020a). However, language like this opened the possibility for individual teams to adopt new protocols depending on their locations throughout the country. This contrasted with Silver's more centralized response that informed teams not to allow travel and suspended all operations for several months. Goodell's response sought to work through the conditions as best as possible in a non-uniform or decentralized manner. This approach was reiterated in the same memo when Goodell notes there are “varying needs of clubs” and that there might be “unique risk factors that individual club employees may face” (Goodell, 2020a, p. 2, posted in Pelissero, 2020a). In a later memo, Goodell notes that while his office might require certain protocols, in the future these practices could be “adapted and supplemented to ensure compliance with any state and local public health requirements” (Goodell, 2020b, p. 2, posted in Schefter, 2020a). Variable language such as this points to a more “a la carte” approach for each individual team, which again challenges the unilateral response communicated by Silver.

Goodell’s more decentralized leadership also was evident in the eventual decision on stadium capacity. On July 27th, only one day before preseason training camps were set to open, Goodell announced in a public memo that an agreement had been made between the NFL and the NFL Players Association (NFLPA), the labor union that represents all professional football athletes. In a memo, Goodell explained that all current health recommendations were to be followed by every team, including guidelines proposed by health experts and CDC officials. Yet, there was one addition to the NFL’s pandemic policy that defied a centralized operating procedure. In one brief sentence, Goodell wrote “state and local health guidelines will help determine whether fans will attend the games” (Goodell, 2020d, para. 4, posted in Kleiman, 2020). This announcement allowed for each of the 32 franchises in the league to choose whatever stadium capacity policy they desired, as long as it fits within local guidelines. Goodell’s communication again directly contradicts the centralized sport crisis leadership of Silver, who only resumed league play after establishing the restrictive, quarantined bubble campus. Goodell’s response to the dominant anecdote established by Silver prioritized moving forward with more agency for individual teams within the organization.

Adjustable Risks

Though the July 27th agreement between the NFLPA and NFL was lengthy and detailed, the results were contrastingly dissimilar to the protocols put in place by Silver. As early as June 7th, Goodell’s sport crisis leadership began to reveal a theme of adopting *adjustable risks* for players, staff, and employees involved. He wrote that despite protocols to diminish risk, “no set of protocols can eliminate the risk of contracting Covid-19, nor ensure that the disease itself will be mild” (Goodell, 2020c, p. 1, posted in Jones, 2020). In a memo to the league on September 29th, Goodell notified the league that players for the Tennessee Titans had tested positive, but that “this is not unexpected . . . there will be players and staff who will test positive during the season” (Goodell, 2020e, p. 1, posted in Schefter, 2020b). Goodell’s response admits there is inherent risk in performing the league as planned, and staff and players would have to navigate that. Rather than having a rigid set of protocols to mitigate risk for *all* teams, Goodell emphasizes adjustability toward risk in a later memo stating,

> Since the beginning of the pandemic, we have acknowledged and planned for the need to adjust and adapt throughout our season. We know that as long as the Covid-19 virus is in our communities that we will have cases in the NFL. (Goodell, 2020f, p. 1, posted in Pelissero, 2020b)

Rather than trying to be risk-averse, the NFL wanted to work through the inherent dangers in an effort to continue as normally as possible. Goodell's communication consistently reiterates that his leadership style will emphasize adjusting to risk rather than actively trying to eliminate it entirely. On November 18th, Goodell explained,

> As we continue through the season, it will likely be necessary to take further steps to address broader conditions . . . we will continue to incorporate our experience and implement enhancements to the protocols and communicate with each of you on a regular basis. (Goodell, 2020g, p. 2, posted in Wilson, 2020)

Terms such as "evolve," "adapt," and "flexibility" dominate the rhetoric within Goodell's public discourse, in turn building a response that tolerates risk and accepts that cases will be a part of the organization's reality. However, one memo offers a deeper understanding or motivation of Goodell's sport crisis leadership and where he emphasizes what really is at risk. In his October 5th memo, Goodell reiterates his encouragement to remain vigilant to the protocols in place. His reasons for doing so are not to mitigate risk to players but rather for more material purposes:

> The consequences of rescheduling or even missing games are obvious. Our fans will be deprived of games. Competitive inequities will be introduced into our season. Players will not be paid for games not played and clubs will similarly suffer financial consequences. (Goodell, 2020f, p. 1, posted in Pelissero, 2020b)

The quote here reveals the underlying interests, priorities, and concerns within Goodell's response. Risks of positive cases will be tolerated, only as long as they do not interfere with revenue. While health and safety of players and staff are mentioned in the abstract across all of Goodell's communication, rarely does it highlight the potential physical risks in the same manner as the financial risks above.

Indecisive (Re)action

In addition to continually adjusting to risk, the rhetoric of Goodell's sport crisis leadership communicates a tendency toward *indecisive reaction* rather than the quick, measured decision-making of Silver. We argue here that Goodell's decision-making can be referred to as a "wait-and-see" approach, often waiting until the last minute to react to the shifting conditions. To illustrate this one only needs to look at the temporal aspect of the planning and implementation of the 2020 NFL season. With the shutdown of facilities in March, Goodell had over six months to plan for a season under a pandemic. Up until kickoff of the first game in September, no one was sure it would happen.

Goodell announced the cancellation of the entire preseason schedule only one week before training and games were supposed to kick off. Moreover, teams were encouraged to stay within their own training facilities during the preseason and socially distance when possible. This recommendation would prove difficult as football is, after all, a full-contact sport played in close proximity to others. Goodell's decision to pursue a full seventeen-week schedule as normal was the most decisive choice of his leadership. Yet, it was during the season when positive cases began spreading across the league that Goodell's indecisive reaction revealed itself once more. In September, several members of the Tennessee Titans tested positive and were put into quarantine protocols. However, members were photographed practicing on a high school field, despite being ordered by the NFL to quarantine and refrain from team activities. It would be weeks before Goodell decided a consequence for this protocol break, opting to fine the team $350,000, but no suspensions. In a league-wide memo, Goodell tries to caution other teams to continue following protocols and offers new adjustments to the already existing protocols:

> Consider holding all meetings virtually, wear masks or shields during practices and walk-throughs, decrease the size of the traveling party, reduce the time spent in lunchrooms and locker rooms, and consult the proximity tracking device information daily to identify areas where your club could eliminate close contacts. (Goodell, 2020e, p. 2, posted in Pelissero, 2020b)

This non-decisive language feels more like *suggestions* rather than convicted choices or instructions for employees to comply with. Goodell's decisions were also questioned when Cam Newton, star quarterback for the New England Patriots, tested positive before a Sunday game. The game was postponed and played through the following day. However, later that week more players who had played in that re-scheduled game ended up testing positive. The lack of consistent administration of quarantine policy and repercussions left many in the public to question the logic of Goodell's policies. Additionally, while players were not required to wear masks while standing on the sidelines, coaches were. Yet, several prime-time games featured coaches who refused to adhere to the policy, forcing Goodell and the league to fine them retroactively (Belson, 2020).

Repeatedly, Goodell's indecisive reactions lacked a consistent rationale. This was seen in the case of postponing and rescheduling games with players testing positive sometimes but not always. In some cases, Goodell's office allowed games to take place, despite pulling players who tested positive off of the field moments before kickoff. It should be noted that Goodell's decision-making ability was partially hindered by the protocols he agreed to with the NFLPA. This agreement allowed for flexibility at all levels of decision-making within the league. For example, per the agreement, clubs were able to decide which level of protocol intensity they wanted to adopt at the beginning of the season. However, in the eleventh week of the season, as cases were rising nationally and within the league, Goodell wrote to teams declaring that "beginning Saturday, November 21, all clubs will conduct their operations under the Intensive Protocols" (Goodell, 2020g, p. 2, posted in Wilson, 2020). Goodell waited nearly three months to require all teams to adopt the more restrictive and risk-averse measures. Which raises the question, if he had the ability to make the executive decision for all teams to adopt the strict guidelines, why wait so long?

Despite themes of decentralized responses, constant adjustment to risk, and indecisive reactions, the NFL completed their season in full. With this feat in mind, one can credit Goodell's sport crisis leadership for reducing the financial hit to the league's overall revenue. Additionally, despite the discordant response, the health of players and staff remained relatively safe. From August 1st through the end of the season, the NFL had only a 0.076 percent positivity rate—"726 infections among 959,860 tests . . . which was far lower than the national average of 6.8% over a similar period" (Seifert, 2021, para. 8). Yet despite this track record, many criticized the league for putting players, personnel, and spectators at risk in the pursuit of profit. While these numbers seem low, we still do not know the long-term effects of Covid-19, and these relatively small numbers do not reflect the physical toll it might have inflicted on individuals. For example, player Ryquell Armstead was hospitalized twice for respiratory issues after testing positive in early August of 2020. He has yet to return to playing football and some speculate if he ever will be able to return (Leonard, 2021). Ultimately, when contrasted with Silver's dominant response, Goodell's discordant response reveals a prioritized interest to secure financial security over the safety of players, staff, and spectators. Or, as sports journalist Bomani Jones pointed out, "Everybody has a financial incentive to do as best as they can in order to keep this thing going" (Harris, 2020, para. 24).

MOVING TOWARD SPORT CRISIS LEADERSHIP PRACTICE

Discordant pandemic responses from the NBA and NFL commissioners highlight the challenges sport crisis leaders face in crisis situations and the myriad of responses leaders may communicate to their stakeholders. This section of the chapter reflects the discordant sport crisis leadership analysis in conjunction with rhetorical leadership practices to consider a path forward for sport crisis leaders. In other words, this section of the chapter considers Silver and Goodell's communication and its implications for the study of leadership and its related practices in the context of crises. In concert with the leadership-as-practice (L-A-P) movement, this chapter attends to the study of leadership (specifically sport crisis leadership) as it "emerges and evolves in concrete social contexts" (Raelin, 2017, p. 219). Undergirded by the argument of leadership as meaning management (Fairhurst & Connaughton, 2014), we consider what communicative practices comprise sport crisis leadership.

Crisis leadership is central to navigating the chaos of crises as leaders help stakeholders to manage uncertainty amidst the catastrophe. From messages of efficacy to messages of renewal, the discourse and actions of leaders during times of crisis has a significant bearing on the outcome, or at minimum, how stakeholders perceive the crisis, organizations, and societies as the crisis unfolds and how stakeholders perceive the new normal that begins to take hold (Ulmer et al., 2019). Leadership is a rather ubiquitous process that has been examined extensively across disciplines, but this chapter directs attention to the work of Fairhurst and colleagues. Fairhurst (2005) advances framing as a linguistic resource for leaders to manage meaning. Communication perspectives of leadership demonstrate a situated, relational ontology where leadership is a rhetorical process of meaning management versus the traditional managerial view of directing or managing people (Fairhurst & Connaughton, 2014; Fairhurst & Sarr, 1996). When leadership is cast as meaning management, the leader acts as the rhetor. Given the move to an applied social construction perspective in communication leadership scholarship (Fairhurst & Grant, 2010), this chapter combines Silver's and Goodell's rhetoric with the communicative practices of framing, narrating, and reflecting on suggesting practice recommendations for sport crisis leaders.

Framing the Crisis Response

Sport crisis leaders should use framing to manage meaning and relationships in their crisis communication. Fairhurst and Sarr (1996) advocate leaders communicating intentionally to frame, or manage meaning, in their interactions. *Framing* is the communicative process that shapes interpretation of message content, relational context between communicators, and the construction of reality (Bateson, 1972; Berger & Luckman, 1966; Fairhurst, 2005). Fairhurst and Sarr (1996) argue that framing stems from language, thought, and forethought, and by forging a union between language and thought in spontaneous interaction, in which rhetors use forethought to control or manage meaning at the moment. Additionally, Fairhurst (2005) explains that the inability or failure to frame may be attributed to poor message design logics. Barbara O'Keefe's work (1988) with message design logics explains how individuals use communication to achieve multiple influence goals. The rhetorical design logic (as opposed to the expressive or conventional design logics) is a complex communication process in which rhetors construct and negotiate their "social selves and situations" by matching and adapting their communication to fit the situation and their goals (Fairhurst, 2005, p. 173).

Applying Fairhurst and Sarr's (1996) framing to sport crisis leadership, sport crisis leaders should simultaneously embrace how their communication transmits information and shapes meaning through intentional communication that merges language, thought, and forethought. Whether using metaphors, narratives, or something else as linguistic framing devices, sports crisis leaders should consider their goals related to the crisis, stakeholder relationships, image (individual and organizational), and crisis recovery/renewal. To illustrate, consider the discordant responses of Silver and Goodell. Goodell missed opportunities for transcendent rhetorical design logics to frame the delayed decision-making and decentralization as *empowering decentralization.* Reframing delays, delegated decisions, and inconsistencies as *empowering decentralization* could have highlighted the positive intentions and outcomes of the NFL's negotiation with the players' union and franchises that led to delayed, decentralized action. This was a missed opportunity to frame as a sport crisis leader.

Narrating the Crisis Response

Narrative is a rhetorical resource sport crisis leaders should harness. In his treatise on the narrative paradigm, Walter Fisher (1985) describes human communicators in terms of their capacity to narrate stories. In reference to crisis communication, Seeger and Sellnow (2016) build on Fisher's work in the narrative paradigm, explaining that crisis narratives function as sensemaking accounts of crises that help fill in knowledge gaps and influence crisis action. Given that the conventional crisis leadership wisdom advocates that leaders are visible, communicate frequently and honestly, and cooperate with stakeholders (Barton, 2008; Ulmer et al., 2019), it logically follows that leaders would use these communication opportunities for good storytelling. To illustrate, reconsider Silver's narration of the first game cancellation and temporary season suspension that followed. Verbally weaving together characters, action, suspense, and timing, Silver constructs a hero narrative. Clarifying the properties of a hero narrative, Seeger and Sellnow (2016) state that hero narratives include "exhibiting self-sacrifice, resoluteness, altruistic behavior, rising to the requirements of the situation, and conferring hero status" (p. 113). While sport crisis leaders need not construct leader-centric narratives casting themselves as heroes, sport crisis leaders can learn from Silver's willingness to tell the NBA's story and do so in a way that fills in knowledge gaps for listeners, provides an account of events, and frames the narrative action and outcome positively.

Reflecting on Crisis Response

Sport crisis leaders have an ethical obligation to lead their organizations and stakeholders to reflect and learn from crises. Fairhurst and Connaughton (2014) introduce reflection as an ethical commitment of leadership practice regarding the push for leaders to "both focus on the opportunities for reflexivity and change in present moments and 're-storying' to affect more ethically and relationally responsive leadership in action" (pp. 21–22). Further clarifying the productive process and outcome of reflection, Ulmer and associates (2019) explain, "By communicating the lessons, leaders enhance safety and prevention, increase an organization's vigilance, and demonstrate its values" (p. 122). The lingering conditions of the coronavirus pandemic at the time of this writing challenge our ability to see long-term reflection by the commissioners. However, we anticipate reflections by a myriad of NBA and NFL stakeholders to emerge and shape future sport crisis leadership practice.

CONCLUSION

In review, this chapter has explored a particular context of discordant pandemic rhetoric—sport crisis communication. As sport and crisis communication continue to expand their research scope and reach, sport crisis communication is a natural intersection of these two subfields. Specifically, this chapter "Discordant Rhetorical Responses: Crisis Communication in Sports Organizations in the COVID-19 Pandemic" extends extant work on sport crisis leadership by analyzing themes within discordant responses of two professional sports organizations in the US with global appeal. The NBA Commissioner Silver's response demonstrated centralization of response, emphasis on caution, and decisive (top-level) action, whereas the NFL Commissioner Goodell's discordant response demonstrated de-centralization of response, adjustment of risks, and indecision or delayed action. Despite frequent communication about health risks and adherence to public health recommendations, Silver's and Goodell's sport crisis leadership rhetoric emphasized discordance in temporal components of decision-making, centralization of decision-making, and tolerance of risk.

With that said, Silver and Goodell faced several notable differences in their COVID-19 crisis contexts. The NBA's season was underway when COVID-19 interrupted play in March 2020, subsequently demanding swift, decisive action. The NFL's 2020 season did not begin until six months after the initial *15 and 30 Days to Slow the Spread* campaigns in the US that shut down the majority of the country, thus enabling Goodell to delay and delegate decision-making. Furthermore, the size of the NBA and NFL teams differ, as do their organizational policies, resources, and structures, which points to many of the dynamics that this study does not analyze by choosing to focus on the direct and mediated statements made by the two commissioners. These noted differences in a pandemic context likely contributed to the discordant anecdotes that ensued.

In response to the discordance, two points are emphasized with regard to sport crisis leadership rhetoric. First, discordance in sport crisis leadership rhetoric was partly attributed to the discord in Silver's and Goodell's rhetorical emphasis on certain motives (e.g., Silver's emphasis on risk aversion through caution and Goodell's emphasis on risk tolerance). However, discordance was likely affected by a number of compounding complexities, including timing. Applying Walter Fisher's work (1985) with narrative as "good reasons" in argumentation, we draw on the principles of fidelity and probability to explain Silver's leadership as rhetorically dominant. Audiences judge "good reasons" based on their "comparison and contrast with prior, accepted stories" (Fisher, 1985, p. 364). Silver's sport crisis leadership anecdote preceded Goodell's, and timing positions audiences to compare the two when judging fidelity and probability. Walter Fisher (1985) explains that fidelity is concerned with whether or not rhetoric seems true, valid, and employs logical structure and reasons, and probability is whether rhetoric is coherent, consistent, and without fallacy. To determine fidelity, the question, "Does the rhetoric ring true?" is asked. Considering fidelity, Silver's themes of centralized, decisive, and quick action effectively resumed NBA play and contained the virus. Considering probability, Silver's accounts are coherent and consistent in his prioritization of caution and central control. Because

Silver's effective rhetoric transpires first, it, therefore, has primacy as audiences compare the NBA and NFL commissioners. Audiences ask the fidelity and probability questions slightly differently: "Does Goodell's rhetoric ring true and cohere with Silver's rhetoric?" Given the discordance highlighted in our analysis, Goodell's leadership becomes the counter of Silver's response and suffers from its temporal ordering.

Second, discordance in the sport crisis leadership opens a dialogue regarding best practices to develop rhetorical resources for future responses. Silver's and Goodell's rhetoric function to "determine future decisions or actions" (Fisher, 1985, p. 362), and SALIENT rhetoric, especially, shape future rhetorical action (Harter & Japp, 2001). Following this strand of reasoning, Silver's response of sport crisis leadership becomes a contextualized model to further study at the intersections of communication, crisis, leadership, and sport, as do the three sport crisis leadership practices—framing, narrating, and reflecting. To advance sport crisis communication studies in conjunction with leadership, continued research is needed to explore how athletes, coaches, managers, teams, organizations, media, fans, and other stakeholders communicatively manage crises disrupting *play* and *business as usual*. "Leadership as the management of meaning expands to all leadership actors (formal or informal leaders, followers or other stakeholders) who can be transformative agents, but also passive receptors of meaning and disciplined products of culture" (Fairhurst & Connaughton, 2014, p. 23). Pandemic conditions presented by the coronavirus demonstrate complex, contested, fluid, and unstable contexts. Further work may explore micro, meso, and macrolevels of crisis communication and how they interpenetrate as leaders in sport contexts engage in crisis planning, decision-making, framing, and recovering.

REFERENCES

Aschburner, S. (2020, October 10). Silver outlines "safe and responsible plan" for NBA comeback. *NBA.com*. Retrieved from https://www.nba.com/news/adam-silver-outlines-safe-and-responsible-plan-nba-comeback

Barton, L. (2008). *Crisis leadership now: A real-world guide to preparing for threats, disaster, sabotage, and scandal.* New York: McGraw Hill.

Bateson, G. (1972). *Steps to an ecology of the mind.* New York: Ballentine.

Belson, K. (2020, October 25). N.F.L. punishes Titans for their handling of coronavirus outbreak. *The New York Times*. Retrieved from https://www.nytimes.com/2020/10/25/sports/football/covid-outbreak-titans-workout.html

Benoit, W. L. (1995). *Accounts, excuses, and apologies: A theory of image restoration.* Albany, NY: State University of New York Press.

Benoit, W. L., & Hanczor, R. S. (1994). The Tonya Harding controversy: An analysis of image restoration strategies. *Communication Quarterly, 42,* 416–433. Doi: 10.1080/01463379409369947

Berger, P., & Luckman, T. L. (1966). *The social construction of knowledge: A treatise on the sociology of knowledge.* New York: Doubleday.

Blaney, J. R., Lippert, L. R., & Smith, S. J. (Eds.). (2013). *Repairing the athlete's image: Studies in sports image restoration.* Lanham, MD: Lexington Books.

Bontemps, T. (2020, June 17). In documents, NBA details coronavirus testing protocols, including 2-week resting period for positive tests. *ESPN*. Retrieved from https://www.espn.com/nba/story/_/id/29321006/in-documents-nba-details-coronavirus-testing-process-orlando-campus-life

Braun, V., & Clarke, V. (2006). Using thematic analysis in psychology. *Qualitative Research in Psychology, 3,* 77–101. Doi: 10.10.1191/1478088706qp063oa

Braun V., & Clarke, V. (2012). Thematic analysis. In H. Cooper (Ed.), *APA handbook of research methods in psychology* (pp. 57–71). Doi: 10.1037/13620–004

Braun, V., & Clarke, V. (2019). Reflecting on reflexive thematic analysis. *Qualitative Research in Sport, Exercise and Health, 11*(4), 589–597. Doi: 10.1080/2159676X.2019.1628806

Brazeal, L. M. (2008). The image repair strategies of Terrell Owens. *Public Relations Review, 34,* 145–150. Doi: 10.1016/j.pubrev.2008.03.021

Brown, N. A., Brown, K. A., & Billings, A. C. (2015). "May no act of ours bring shame": Fan-enacted crisis communication surrounding the Penn State sex abuse scandal. *Communication & Sport, 3*(3), 288–311. Doi: 10.1177/2167479513514387

Centers for Disease Control and Prevention. (2021, January 15). CDC COVID data tracker. Retrieved from https://covid.cdc.gov/covid-data-tracker/#cases_casesper100klast7days

Coombs, W. T., & Holladay, S. J. (2008). Comparing apology to equivalent crisis response strategies: Clarifying apology's role and value in crisis communication. *Public Relations Review, 34*(3), 252–257. Doi: 10.1016/j.ubrev.2008.04.001

Coombs, W. T. (2018). Athlete reputational crises: One point for linking—situational crisis communication theory and sports crises. In A. C. Billings, W. T. Coombs, & K. A. Brown (Eds.), *Reputational challenges in sport: Theory and application* (pp. 13–24). New York: Routledge.

Debenedetti, G. (2020, March 12). Obama's Ebola Czar on how Trump has bungled coronavirus response. *Intelligencer.* Retrieved from https://nymag.com/intelligencer/2020/03/obamas-ebola-czar-on-how-trump-bungled-coronavirus-response.html

Delante, N. (2020). Classroom teaching as intercultural communication phenomenon: A thematic analysis of a foreign teacher's rhetorical practices as communication dynamic. *Journal of Intercultural Communication Research, 49*(6), 536–568. Doi: 10.1080/17475759.2020.1790406

de Blasio, B. [@NYCMayor]. (2020, March, 17). *We wish them a speedy recovery. But, with all due respect, an entire NBA team should NOT get tested for* [Tweet] Twitter. https://twitter.com/NYCMayor/status/1240029424394829829?s=20

DiFiori, J. P., Green, G., Meeuwisse, W., Putukian, M., Solomon, G. S., & Sills, A. (2021). Return to sport for North American professional sport leagues in the context of COVID-19. *British Journal of Sports Medicine, 55,* 417–421. Doi: 10.1136/bjsports-2020–103227

Fairhurst, G. T. (2005). Reframing the art of framing: Problems and prospects for leadership. *Leadership, 1*(2), 165–185. Doi: 10.1177.1742715005051857

Fairhurst, G. T., & Connaughton, S. L. (2014). Leadership: A communicative perspective. *Leadership, 10*(1), 7–35. Doi: 10.1177/1742715013509396

Fairhurst, G. T., & Grant, D. (2010). The social construction of leadership: A sailing guide. *Management Communication Quarterly, 24,* 171–210. Retrieved from https://doi.org/10.1177/0893318909359697

Fairhurst, G. T., & Sarr, R. A. (1996). *The art of framing.* San Francisco: Jossey-Bass.

Farhi, P. (2010). Lost in the woods. *American Journalism Review, 32(1),* 14–19.

Fisher, W. R. (1985). The narrative paradigm: An elaboration. *Communication Monographs, 52*(4), 347–367. Retrieved from https://doi.org/10.1080/03637758509376117

Fortunato, J. (2008). Restoring a reputation: The Duke University lacrosse scandal. *Public Relations Review, 34,* 116–123. Doi: 10.1016/j.pubrev.2008.03.006

Goodell, R. (2020a, April 6). Memorandum: Status of club facilities/2020, NFL Draft [Tweet; attached photo]. *NFL.* Retrieved from https://twitter.com/TomPelissero/status/1247230356354367494

Goodell, R. (2020b, May 6). Memorandum: Public comment on 2020 season/reopening of club facilities [Tweet; attached photo]. *NFL.* Retrieved from https://twitter.com/AdamSchefter/status/1258187503313575936

Goodell, R. (2020c, June 7). Memorandum: Protocols for player return to club facility. [Tweet; attached photo]. *NFL.* Retrieved from https://twitter.com/jjones9/status/1270016041716977665

Goodell, R. (2020d, July 27). Public memo. *NFL.* [Tweet; attached photo]. Retrieved from https://twitter.com/NFL_DovKleiman/status/1287814503921528832

Goodell, R. (2020e, September 29). Memorandum: Covid-19 positives at Tennessee Titans. [Tweet; attached photo]. *NFL.* Retrieved from https://twitter.com/adamschefter/status/1311021028139827205

Goodell, R. (2020f, October 5). Memorandum: Covid-19 protocol compliance. [Tweet; attached photo]. *NFL.* Retrieved from https://twitter.com/tompelissero/status/1313207707512590341?lang=en

Goodell, R. (2020g, November 18). Memorandum: Enhanced Covid-19 protocol. [Tweet; attached photo]. *NFL.* Retrieved from https://twitter.com/aaronwilson_nfl/status/1329161732770701312

Harker, J. L., & Saffer, A. J. (2018). Mapping a subfield's sociology of science: A 25-year network and bibliometric analysis of the knowledge construction of sports crisis communication. *Journal of Sport and Social Issues, 42*(5), 369–392. Doi: 10.1177/0193723518790011

Harris, M. (2020, December 7). How did the NFL get into this mess? *Slate Magazine.* Retrieved from https://slate.com/culture/2020/12/nfl-coronavirus-outbreaks-bomani-jones-explains.html

Harter, L. M., & Japp, P. M. (2001). Technology as the representative anecdote in popular discourses of health and medicine. *Health Communication, 13*(4), 409–425. Retrieved from https://doi.org/10.1207/s15327027hc1304_04

Herbert, J. (2020, March 19). Coronavirus: All of the unanswered questions for Adam Silver, NBA amid the COVID-19 shutdown. *CBSSports.com*. Retrieved from https://www.cbssports.com/nba/news/coronavirus-all-of-the-unanswered-questions-for-adam-silver-nba-amid-the-covid-19-shutdown/

Hermann, C. F. (1963). Some consequences of crisis which limit the viability of organizations. *Administrative Science Quarterly, 8*(1), 61–82.

Holeyman, M. (2020, April 24). This doctor survived Ebola: This is her message on COVID-19. *Thomas Reuters Foundation.* Retrieved from https://news.trust.org/item.20200424141138-zqaif

Ishak, A. W. (2017). Communication in sports teams: A review. *Communication Research Trends, 36*(4), 4–38. Retrieved from http://cscc.scu.edu/trends/v36/CRT_v36_n4_December_2017.pdf

Jackson, J., & Thaker, J. (2021). Letting the team down? Examining sport fans reactions to Aaron Smith's "toilet tryst" on social media. *Communication Research and Practice, 7*(2), 148–172. Doi: 10.1080/22041451.2021.1905942

Jerome, A. M. (2008). Toward prescription: Testing the rhetoric of atonement's applicability in the athletic arena. *Public Relations Review, 34,* 124–134. Doi: 10.1016/j.pubrev.2008.03.007

Jones, J. [@jjones9]. (2020, June 8). *Memo to NFL teams from Roger Goodell on a player return to team facilities. No date is given here but* [Tweet; attached photo]. Twitter. https://twitter.com/jjones9/status/1270016041716977665

Kleiman, D. [@NFL_DovKleiman]. (2020, July 27). *Letter from Roger Goodell* [Tweet; attached photo]. Twitter.https://twitter.com/NFL_DovKleiman/status/1287814503921528832

Leonard, P. (2021, June 26). NFL notes: Giants cut Ryquell Armstead, throwback helmets return, Xavier McKinney on the Eagles' tank. *nydailynews.com*. Retrieved from https://www.nydailynews.com/sports/football/giants/ny-sunday-nfl-notes-20210626-wvaq6b4utve6jn3svo32ebvkdm-story.html

Lombardo, J. (2020, October 19). NBA preserved $1.5B in revenue at Disney, but losses are steep. *Sports Business Journal*. Retrieved from https://www.sportsbusinessjournal.com/Journal/Issues/2020/10/19/Leagues-and-Governing-Bodies/NBA-bubble.aspx

Mahoney, B. (2020, October 10). NBA tells teams to plan for empty arenas; LeBron says no way. *NBA.com*. Retrieved from https://www.nba.com/news/coronavirus-lebron-wont-play-empty-arenas

Meng, J., & Pan, P. (2013). Revisiting image-restoration strategies: An integrated case study of three athlete sex scandals in sports news. *International Journal of Sport Communication, 6*(1), 87–100. Retrieved from https://doi.org/10.1123/ijsc.6.1.87

Newson, M. (2019). Football, fan violence, and identity fusion. *International Review for the Sociology of Sport, 54*(4), 431–444. Doi: 10.1177/1012690217731293

Oxner, R. (2020, October 12). Lakers win NBA finals; No coronavirus cases reported in bubble. *NPR*. Retrieved from https://www.npr.org/2020/10/12/923064484/lakers-win-nba-finals-no-coronavirus-cases-reported-in-bubble

O'Keefe, B. J. (1988). The logic of message design: Individual differences in reasoning about communication. *Communication Monographs, 55,* 10–103.

Partridge-Hicks, S. (2020, September 11). 5 countries that are getting COVID-19 responses right. *Global Citizen.* Retrieved from https://www.globalcitizen.org/en/content/countries-with-best-covid-responses/

Pedersen, P. M. (Ed.). (2013). *Routledge handbook of sport communication.* New York: Routledge.

Pelissero, T. [@TomPelissero]. (2020a, April 6). *NFL commissioner Roger Goodell just informed clubs in a memo that club facilities will remain closed indefinitely and the league* [Tweet; attached photo]. Twitter. https://twitter.com/tompelissero/status/1247230356354367494?lang=en

Pelissero, T. [@TomPelissero]. (2020b, October 5). *NFL Commissioner Roger Goodell with a pointes message to clubs on COVID-19 protocols: "Simply put, compliance is mandatory"* [Tweet; attached photo]. Twitter. https://twitter.com/tompelissero/status/1313207707512590341?lang=en

ProFootballTalk. [@ProFootballTalk]. (2020, March 22). *Here's Roger Goodell's full March 19 letter to all NFL employees regarding COVID-19* [Tweet; attached link to article]. Twitter. https://twitter.com/ProFootballTalk/status/1241733292933726213

Raelin, J. A. (2017). Leadership-as-practice: Theory and application—An editor's reflection. *Leadership, 13*(2), 215–221. Doi: 10.1177/1742715017702273

Reynolds, T. (2020a, March 20). NBA shuttering facilities as more teams face positive tests. *NBA.com*. Retrieved from https://www.nba.com/news/nba-shuttering-facilities-more-teams-face-positive-tests

Reynolds, T. (2020b, October 10). NBA players staying up-to-date on coronavirus crisis. *NBA.com*. Retrieved from https://www.nba.com/news/nba-coronavirus-memo-avoid-high-fives

Schefter, A. [@AdamSchefter]. (2020a, May 7). *Memo that went today from Roger Goodell to team presidents and executives regarding the 2020 season and the reopening of* [Tweet; attached photo]. Twitter. https://twitter.com/AdamSchefter/status/1258187503313575936

Schefter, A. [@AdamSchefter]. (2020b, September 29). *Email that NFL commissioner Roger Goodell sent today to all team Presidents and Executives.* [Tweet; attached photo]. Twitter. https://twitter.com/adamschefter/status/1311021028139827205

Sedano, M. V. (1980). Chicanismo: A rhetorical analysis of themes and images of selected poetry from the Chicano Movement. *Western Journal of Speech Communication, 44*(3), 177–190.

Seeger, M. W., & Sellnow, T. L. (2016). *Narratives of crisis: Telling stories of ruin and renewal.* Stanford, CA: Stanford University Press.

Seifert, K. (2021, February 12). How the NFL navigated COVID-19 this season: 959,860 tests, $100 million and zero cancellations. *ESPN*. Retrieved from https://www.espn.com/nfl/story/_/id/30781978/how-nfl-navigated-covid-19-season-959860-tests-100-million-zero-cancellations

Shelburne, R. (2020, March 19). How the NBA moved so quickly on coronavirus testing. *ESPN*. Retrieved from https://www.espn.com/nba/story/_/id/28925716/how-nba-moved-quickly-coronavirus-testing

Spaaij, R. (2016). Terrorism and security at the Olympics: Empirical trends and evolving research agendas. *The International Journal of the History of Sport, 33*(4), 451–468. Doi: 10.1080/09523367.2015.1136290

Spradley, R. T. (2017). Crisis communication in organizations. *The International Encyclopedia of Organizational Communication*. Doi: 10.1002/9781118955567.wbieoc050

Ulmer, R. R., Sellnow, T. L., & Seeger, M. W. (2019). *Effective crisis communication: Moving from crisis to opportunity* (4th ed.). Thousand Oaks, CA: Sage.

Walsh, J., & McAllister-Spooner, S. M. (2011). Analysis of the image repair discourse in the Michael Phelps controversy. *Public Relations Review, 37*(2), 157–162. Doi: 10.1016/j.pubrev.2011.01.001.

Wicker, P., Filo, K., & Cuskelly, G. (2013). Organizational resilience of community sport clubs impacted by natural disasters. *Journal of Sport Management, 27*(6), 510–525. Doi: 10.1123/jsm.27.6.510

Wilson, A. [@AaronWilson_NFL]. (2020, November 18). *NFL memo from Roger Goodell on enhanced protocols instituted for all 32 teams* [Tweet; attached photo]. Twitter. https://twitter.com/aaronwilson_nfl/status/1329161732770701312

Zillgitt, J., & Medina, M. (2021, March 12). Inside the night the NBA postponed its season. *USA Today*. Retrieved from https://www.usatoday.com/in-depth/sports/nba/2021/03/11/nba-shutdown-inside-look-night-nba-postponed-their-season/4637550001/

Zompetti, J. P. (2019). Rhetorical incivility in the Twittersphere: A comparative thematic analysis of Clinton and Trump's Tweets during and after the 2016 presidential election. *Journal of Contemporary Rhetoric, 9*(1–2), 29–54. Retrieved from http://contemporaryrhetoric.com/wp-content/uploads/2019/02/Zompetti9_1_2_3.pdf

Chapter Seven

Misinformation, Scandalization, and the *Trump Show*

Audience Responses to President Trump's Pandemic Narrative

Kristjan Kikerpill

At the time of writing, the COVID-19 pandemic has claimed the lives of more than four million people globally and six hundred thousand in the United States (Worldometer, 2021). Similar to the flu pandemic of 1918, the emergence and spread of COVID-19 sent world communities scrambling for solutions (Morens et al., 2021). The mitigation and management of any large-scale crisis relies heavily on communication (Hansson et al., 2020), particularly on communication from governments and leadership (Kim & Kreps, 2020; Liu et al., 2020). In health crises, best practices recommend quickly filling any information vacuums, being frank and telling the truth, as well as avoiding over-assuring and speculation (Covello, 2003).

Following a debacle at a pandemic briefing in late April 2020, which included suggestions of injecting bleach and the use of light "inside of the body" for the purpose of countering the effects of COVID-19 (BBC, 2020, para. 11), President Donald J. Trump (DT) briefly stayed out of the public eye. According to DT, the regular briefings were "not worth the time and effort" (Aratani, 2020, para. 2). Upon continuing with the pandemic briefings in July (Liptak, 2020)—partly because previous pandemic briefings had "record numbers watching" (Bump, 2020, para. 4)—the 45th President of the United States also gave two interviews to representatives of two very different media establishments. The first interview was carried out by Christopher Wallace for Fox News and aired on July 19, 2020 [YouTube Video "President

Trump goes one-on-one with Chris Wallace"] (Fox News, 2020a), and the second by Jonathan Swan for Axios on HBO, which aired on August 3, 2020 [YouTube Video "AXIOS on HBO: President Trump Exclusive Interview (Full Episode) | HBO"] (Axios on HBO, 2020[1]; Melmax7, 2020). Reporters and commentators found plenty of highlight-reel transgressions in both interviews (Holpuch, 2020; Schwartz, 2020). However, one phrase, which DT uttered in both interviews when responding to questions about the high number of infection cases and deaths from the COVID-19 virus in the United States, stands out: "it is what it is" (Fox News, 2020b, para. 58; Schwartz, 2020, para. 7; Rev, 2020, 07:27). This phrase provided the impetus for researching and writing this chapter, "Misinformation, Scandalization, and the Trump Show: Audience Responses to President Trump's Pandemic Narrative," for three interconnected reasons.

Firstly, DT's regular briefings went on hiatus because these were seen as hurting DT politically (Baker & Haberman, 2020) and returned in the hopes that the resumption of briefings would bolster DT's approval (Bump, 2020) because efforts to "play down the seriousness of the continuing pandemic" were not successful (Baker & Haberman, 2020, para. 15). Given DT's well-documented adversarial relationship with facts and the truth (Kessler et al., 2020), continued dissemination of misinformation and misleading claims by DT were only to be expected. At the time of the interview with Christopher Wallace in July 2020, two-thirds of Americans did not trust the information DT provided with respect to the pandemic (Quinnipiac University, 2020). Hence, it would be difficult to suggest that the only purpose of DT's public pandemic briefings was the provision of important crisis information. For instance, Bump (2020) pointed out that DT himself seemed most concerned about getting people to watch and added that "people are a lot more interested in watching car crashes than smoothly running highways" (para. 17).

Secondly, openly anticipating mishaps whenever DT stood in front of a camera or had a microphone pointed towards him was a strong indication that DT's public appearances carried entertainment value, even where this came in the form of *schadenfreude*, that is, enjoyment obtained from the misfortune of others (see Foreman, 2020). According to Kendzior (2020), the Trump administration was "like a reality show featuring villains from every major political scandal of the past forty years" (p. 7). Thus, while surveys suggested that the American people considered DT's pandemic information briefings untrustworthy, these public appearances still never failed to draw a crowd. The aforementioned observation inevitably begs the question of what exactly the audiences of DT's public appearances were reacting to.

Thirdly, in the era of post-truth politics, facts are less important than appeals to emotion when it comes to capturing an audience (e.g., Tsipursky, 2017). In addition to being the staple of any politician's diet, audiences are also the lifeblood of the media—a lack of viewers spells lower ratings and decreased revenues. As president, DT was notorious for creating media feedback loops, that is, first absorbing news coverage about himself, then commenting furiously on social media about what he saw and heard, and, by doing so, generating a slew of media stories (Miroff, 2018, p. 273). What the media gained from such feedback loops was perhaps best summarized by former CBS executive chairman Leslie Moonves's 2016 remark about DT's candidacy: "It may not be good for America, but it's damn good for CBS" (Bond, 2016, para. 3).

Health crises impose a burden on the media to keep the public constantly informed (Ogbodo et al., 2020), which explains the prevalence of the COVID-19 pandemic as a news topic (Zuckerman, 2020). However, it does not explain why the media would provide extensive coverage of and the audience would tune in to listen to someone who is more likely to misinform than inform. That is, unless certain coverage was less about informing and more about scandalizing, journalists trying to persuade the public of the existence of a scandal with the aim of eliciting public outrage (Geiß, 2017; Graßl et al., 2019), and perpetuating the so-called *Trump Show*. Since the meaning of messages, and the acceptance or rejection of messages, is ultimately determined by recipients (e.g., Hall, 1973), only audience responses can clarify the aforementioned matter.

Thus, by analyzing audience responses to former President Trump's pandemic narrative as captured in the interviews conducted by Christopher Wallace and Jonathan Swan, this chapter seeks answers to the following: (1) what were the audience members reacting to as they watched the interviews? and (2) whether, based on audience responses, there is cause to consider these interviews as instances of (dark) entertainment instead of crisis communication.

This chapter is structured with a brief overview of the social context and theoretical considerations for the study followed by a description of the methods for data collection and analysis. Findings will then be presented, which challenge the status of DT's interview appearances as crisis communication, and the discussion will follow.

THEORETICAL BACKGROUND

From Crisis Communication to the *Trump Show* Hiatus

Disasters and crises that take a toll on human life are inherently characterized by change, high levels of uncertainty, and interactive complexity (Reynolds & Quinn, 2008; Seeger et al., 2003). As the management and mitigation of crises relies heavily on communication, both the resilience of technical infrastructure and the veracity of information being disseminated are crucial (Hansson et al., 2020). While comparisons of devastating health-related disasters always warrant caution, there are important aspects that the 1918 influenza pandemic, that is, the deadliest pandemic to date (Amenabar, 2020), and the COVID-19 pandemic share. Although World War I placed certain restrictions on what reporters could publish (Halsey, 2018), the vastly expanded mass-media network of the early twentieth century meant that the influenza pandemic was played out in a very public manner (Tomes, 2010). As Jordan (1927) remarked,

> . . . rarely if ever before in the annals of medicine has a manifestation of epidemic disease been studied by numerous observers with so much ardor and reported with so much fullness as was the epidemic—perhaps the greatest of all influenza epidemics—of 1918. (p. 3)

On a less inspired note, editors of the time had also learned from previous experience that disease stories sold newspapers (Tomes, 2010). Thus, while the COVID-19 virus itself was new, the suddenly increased information needs of people wanting to know more about the virus' spread, effects, and consequences were not.

In fact, the information dissemination response accompanying COVID-19 was so intense, it created an infodemic, i.e., an overabundance of information, both online and offline (World Health Organization, 2020). The pandemic-specific information disorder involved the creation and consumption of false claims, misleading statements, false rumors, and conspiracy theories (Hansson et al., 2021), and even aided the exploitation of the pandemic for criminal gains (Kikerpill & Siibak, 2021). The complexity of the modern information ecosystem (e.g., Yang et al., 2021) and the rapid horizontal spread of information (Reynolds & Quinn, 2008) make it very difficult to ensure that the guidance people receive is factually correct.

Alongside social resilience, government responses often determine the scope, magnitude, and impact that crises have on society (Mizrahi et al., 2021). The limelight is placed on the role governments and leadership play in managing and mitigating crises (Liu et al., 2020) and can improve trust in government if the crisis is managed well (Goldfinch et al., 2021). A checklist of best practices for health risk and crisis communication proposed by Covello (2003) invites responsible actors to, among other things, be truthful, honest, frank, and open when communicating, as well as to communicate clearly and with compassion. Reynolds and Quinn (2008) further stress that the ability of response officials is "to communicate in a way that connects with those listening" which "may mean the difference between life and death for some people" (p. 13S) because it impacts whether people choose to follow the provided guidance.

Hence, to create order amid the COVID-19 information chaos and provide the public what they yearned for, DT's administration continued the previously abandoned regular information briefings in March 2020 (Baker & Haberman, 2020). However, an analysis of the White House pandemic briefings from March 9th to mid-April 2020 (Peters et al., 2020) suggested that self-regard, credit-taking, and "the audacious rewriting of history to cast himself as the hero of the pandemic rather than the president who was slow to respond" (para. 4) were the defining features of DT's speeches. The briefings were further described as a "daily worship session" for DT (Feinberg, 2020, para. 10), including numerous exaggerations and falsehoods in the information communicated (Peters et al., 2020). Essentially, characterizations of the March–April pandemic briefings read as the polar opposite of what previous research recommends regarding health risk and crisis communication (Covello, 2003; Reynolds & Quinn, 2008). Even so, DT himself seemed satisfied with the process because drawing an average audience of 8.5 million viewers on cable news rivaled the viewership of the season finale of *The Bachelor* (Grynbaum, 2020). Ultimately, DT's violation of the recommendation to avoid speculation in crisis communication (see Covello, 2003) was the reason for calling off the briefings in April, that is, following an aggressive pushback on DT's suggestion that ingesting or injecting disinfectant such as bleach may counter the virus (Baker & Haberman, 2020).

THE POST-HIATUS TRUMP SHOW AND (DARK) ENTERTAINMENT

In July 2020, DT announced the resumption of the daily briefings (Liptak, 2020). With respect to the two interviews analyzed in this chapter, the aforementioned announcement followed the Christopher Wallace interview (aired July 19, 2020) and preceded the recording and airing of the Jonathan Swan interview. Considering that, as president, DT had always been energetic in his efforts to bait the media into creating feedback loops (Miroff, 2018), the return of the so-called *Trump Show* was not unexpected.

Knowing that DT was prone to disseminating misinformation, concerns over the coverage of his appearances dated back to DT's election campaign in 2016 (Grynbaum, 2016). The major difference in 2020 was the contextual backdrop of the COVID-19 pandemic, that is, what had mostly been a secluded discussion among media ethicists now had to take into account that "lives are at risk" (Grynbaum, 2020, para. 7). DT's use of social media, and the media establishment in general, played on the fact that "presidential utterances occupy a special category" (Grynbaum, 2020, para. 10) in American political communication. In other words, DT's communications were shaped around and by identity logic rather than information logic (Jensen, 2018), given that information is far more fleeting than an identity.

The sharp partisan divides in the U.S., including a media that has historically aligned along either Democrat or Republican party lines (Jensen, 2018; Sheppard, 2008), are well-established (Mason, 2018). With respect to understanding American political behavior, previous research suggests a "primacy of a politicized identity over information cues" (Sample et al., 2020, p. 6). Thus, the identity of a speaker takes precedence over the content of utterances. The significance of DT's (social) media presence is further elevated by an understanding that, in online communications, "identity can be a shared feeling" (Zaharna, 2018, p. 60, as cited in Sample et al., 2020, p. 6). Much like the thesis on effective crisis communication (Reynolds & Quinn, 2008), current political discourse cannot afford to underestimate the importance of affect and emotions, particularly the intensity of feelings. In fact, part of DT's popular success was predicated on the notion that DT did "not allow the facts of a situation to interfere with the effectiveness of his emotional appeals" (Miller, 2019, p. 195).

Hence, while access to accurate information has been considered to be a crucial quantity for voters for the purpose of making "correct" decisions (Jensen, 2018, p. 117), and the importance of rhetoric to play an increased accessory role where information costs are high, for example, when information is hard to obtain or difficult to understand without expert knowledge (Posner, 1995, as cited in Miller, 2019), none of this seems to apply to DT's communications (Miller, 2019). Furthermore, intentionally shaping communications based on feelings, speaker-audience identity as well as speculation, which lead to misinformation scandals such as the disinfectant suggestion (Baker & Haberman, 2020), may not necessarily spell trouble for the speaker (Engell, 2005, as cited in Vorberg & Zeitler, 2019).

Therefore, it is important to acknowledge that the media has played a significant role in propping up the controversial star of DT since the 1980s (Kendzior, 2020). Vorberg and Zeitler (2019) established that low moral expectations towards a political figure, for example, former President Trump, can diminish how transgressions grow or fail to grow into public outrage. The scandalization of mild transgressions may lead to lower trust in the news media but has not been found to inevitably lead to lower levels of political trust (Graßl et al., 2019). In effect, this suggests that the news media can—subdued ethics-based considerations aside (see Grynbaum, 2016)—continue scandalization practices if the object of scandalization, for example, another misinformation-filled public appearance of DT, can be passed off as a severe transgression. On the other end, the political figure may not be harmed by the scandal (Graßl et al., 2019), especially if the figure is well-known from television and moral expectations were not high (Vorberg & Zeitler, 2019), and even gain from it (Engell, 2005, as cited in Vorberg & Zeitler, 2019). Since DT's pandemic information was not found to be trustworthy overall (Quinnipiac University, 2020) and DT often spread false claims during the regular pre-hiatus White House pandemic briefings (Peters, Plott, & Haberman, 2020), the continued coverage must have provided some other value, for example, entertainment value.

By now, entertainment has become deeply engrained into traditionally non-entertainment offerings (see Dobni, 2007; Sayre & King, 2003) including the news or "infotainment" (Brants, 1998), and *schadenfreude*-based entertainment is an increasingly common occurrence (Kuipers, 2014). Therefore, any missteps by actors may only add to the entertainment value from the perspective of the benefit component of entertainment (see Dobni, 2007), that is, what the audience perceives to gain from consuming a particular instance of entertainment. However, given that the interpretive backdrop of DT's post-hiatus media blunders (Holpuch, 2020; Schwartz, 2020) was a deadly pandemic, the type of entertainment value gained from it can only be described as coming from what I call dark entertainment.

Conceptually, dark entertainment may be said to be the evil sibling of boilerplate *schadenfreude*-entertainment, for example, *Candid Camera*, blooper TV, and reality TV (Clissold, 2004; Kuipers, 2014). Kuipers (2014, p. 270) explains that *schadenfreude*-based entertainment uses various strategies to neutralize the potential offensiveness of the genre, including distancing, targeting the rich and famous, punishing people who cave in to temptation, or emphasizing people's deservingness (see also Feather, 2014). Where *America's Funniest Home Videos* is an example of common or regular *schadenfreude*-entertainment, the controversial video series *Bumfights* (see Stahl, 2018, para. 22), which depicted "drunk bums beating each other silly," must act as the archetype for dark entertainment. Unlike violent sports which may be controversial but are separately sanctioned (see Guttman, 1998), the authors of *Bumfights* sourced their material and fashioned it into entertainment by exploiting human suffering. An event-proper, for example, a fight between homeless men, can be likened to violent sports only where the reality of an acute social context is suppressed or ignored. In other words, while the entertainment value in dark entertainment derives from an event-proper that is likened to other similar events, the viewer is to concurrently suppress or ignore the backdrop of severe social issues that gave significance to the (*schadenfreude*-) event.

In this chapter, I use the concept of dark entertainment to clearly mark the context that resides behind the potentially *schadenfreude*-inducing, but to some extent expected, communicative mishaps of DT. Thus, DT's interviews with Christopher Wallace and Jonathan Swan primarily act as the narrative vehicles between the devastating human suffering entailed by the COVID-19 pandemic and audience responses to DT's version of crisis management and communication.

DATA AND METHODS

Within less than a month's span, Donald Trump participated in two landmark interviews—first with Chris Wallace for Fox News on July 19, 2020, and with Jonathan Swan for Axios on HBO, which aired August 3, 2020. In search of reactions to DT's often controversial utterances, comments posted to the videos of the two interviews were collected from YouTube for the Fox News interview [YouTube Video "President Trump goes one-on-one with Chris Wallace"] (Fox News, 2020a) (hereinafter also: Trump/Wallace interview) and the Axios on HBO interview [YouTube Video "AXIOS on HBO: President Trump Exclusive Interview (Full Episode) | HBO"] (Axios on HBO, 2020; Melmax7, 2020). (hereinafter also: Trump/Swan interview).

The first interview was for Fox News with Christopher Wallace, and the YouTube video of the interview had N=107,341 comments at the time of collection (Trump/Wallace interview, Fox News, 2020a). The second interview was with Jonathan Swan for Axios on HBO, and the video had N=68,641 comments on YouTube (Trump/Swan interview, Axios on HBO, 2020). After their initial airing, the chosen interviews received extensive media coverage, in particular for certain controversial utterances made by DT (Holpuch, 2020; Schwartz, 2020). Given the number of comments submitted to the interviews on YouTube, supporters and detractors holding strong views were assumed to populate the comment section with arguments both for and against the actions of DT and his administration during the pandemic. Hence, determining whether such commentators had presented their views—positive or negative—required carrying out a sentiment analysis of the submitted comments. I used the Valence Aware Dictionary for sEntiment Reasoning (VADER) sentiment analyzer (Hutto & Gilbert, 2014) to obtain initial polarity values for the comments. The use of the VADER analyzer is justified because YouTube comments resemble social media texts, and the analyzer takes account of aspects such as capitalization and punctuation in determining the intensity of the polarity of a text. Following the initial sentiment assessment where obtained polarity values can range between -1 and 1, thresholds were set for both extremely negative comments (polarity $<=-0.90$) and extremely positive comments (polarity$>=$ 0.90). Comments with polarity values within the imposed ranges were extracted, resulting in N(negative)=2179 and

N(positive)=1744 for the Fox News interview, and N(negative)=1084 and N(positive)=834 for the Axios on HBO interview.

In addition, random samples (N=200) were extracted from each sub-set of comments with extreme polarities (four subsets, i.e., negative and positive from each interview) for subsequent qualitative analysis and verification. Further, following the principle of qualitative text analysis (Kuckartz, 2019; see also Schreier, 2014), open coding of the texts (N=800) was performed on the comment level, that is, one comment formed a unit of analysis. The qualitative analysis was further justified due to comments such as: "My 13-year-old daughter could handle pressure better than this joke of a President! Who uses words like best, wonderful, & greatest—when it comes to people dying from this pandemic?" (User A, comment on Trump/Wallace interview, July 20, 2020). It is obvious that the comment was meant as a snipe against DT, but the inclusion of "best," "wonderful," and "greatest" skews the sentiment towards positive. Thus, subsequent data analysis had to take into account DT's specific manner of self-expression, that is, the excessive use of superlatives like "greatest," and audience members' frequent choice to mimic this, for instance: "Lots of people, good people, they call me, and they say—and these people know what they're talking about—they say they love pizza. They love me, nobody has done more for pizza than me" (User B, comment on Trump/Swan interview, August 4, 2020).

Therefore, comments were manually analyzed to assign a primary descriptor. Four major categories emerged from the coding, namely "supporting," "opposing," "mockery," and "neutral." Support and opposition were labeled with respect to DT, while the "mockery" label was used in cases where sarcasm or satire was directed at DT or exchanged between audience members of diverging views. Comments coded as "neutral" were primarily those that pertained to the actions of the interviewers, but also comments that had no particular bearing for the analysis, e.g., religion-themed comments not directly addressing the interview.

FINDINGS

The results of the coding yielded an almost even split between commentators expressing support for DT (149 of 800 comments, or 18.6 percent) and those expressing some form of opposition towards DT's utterances or behavior (152 of 800 comments, or 19 percent). The largest share of comments was coded as "neutral" (31.9 percent), which included comments from people outside the U.S., comments addressing some aspect or action of the interviewers rather than DT, and comments exchanged between commentators, that is, replies to previous comments. Nevertheless, an important phenomenon emerged within the "neutral" category in the form of expressions of implicit support and opposition as commentators assessed the interviewers' performance, including the entire interaction between DT and the interviewer. There were 244 comments (30.5 percent) coded as "mockery," primarily comprising sarcastic or hostile outbursts towards DT, or exchanged between audience members with diverging views.

Explicitly and Implicitly in Support of Donald Trump

Comments posted in support of Donald Trump were predominantly brief and unambiguous in nature, for instance: "Great job President Trump! God continue to bless you, your family, administration, and continue to strengthen you, you are BEST POTUS EVER! THANK YOU FOR HANGING ON STRONG!!! TRUMP 2020–2024" (User C, comment on Trump/Wallace interview, July 20, 2020). A common characteristic of supportive comments was the inclusion of "2024" or other references in hopes of DT being re-elected. Furthermore, many comments that tried to lift DT up, also attempted to belittle current President Joseph R. Biden:

> If you were really confident about your soul saving candidate Joe Biden you would not be reduced to character assassination of another person as your campaign strategy. It shows how weak and cowardly you are. Here is a suggestion: Next time get a candidate that can complete one sentence without losing their train of thought. (User D, comment on Trump/Wallace interview, July 20, 2020)

In general, commentators supporting DT spent less time addressing the substance of DT's utterances about the ongoing COVID-19 pandemic but focused more on the (then) upcoming presidential election. In that context, DT's personal reappearance in the media was also welcomed by supporters:

> This was great. It was so refreshing to hear Trump speak, instead of some slanderous interpretation by the media. [. . .]. (User E, comment on Trump/Wallace interview, July 20, 2020)
>
> This is one of President Trump's greatest interviews, loved every bit of it. He is forthright and honest about Covid-19, cases are up cause the US has the best testing. (User F, comment on Trump/Wallace interview, July 20, 2020)

Thus, hearing directly from DT was important for those supportive of the former president, even where it reflected the misconception that the absolute number of COVID-19 infections is somehow determined by the amount of testing performed. Moreover, praise for DT was not only expressed in an explicit manner but also appeared as attacks against the interviewers, that is, as challenges against an adversary who dares to doubt or fact-check DT, for example:

> Swan is an obvious hate Trump democrat activist POSING as a journalist. Swan embarrassed himself with his outrageous rudeness and disrespect for the President. He constantly interrupted Trump and interjected his own OPINIONS on the issues. Trump effectively exposed Swan's nonsense and had to educate him. Trump schooled him well! (User G, comment on Trump/Swan interview, August 4, 2020)
>
> Chris Wallace is so biased, rude, condescending, and disrespectful. Don't do an interview if you can't act like a professional journalist. Pathetic. You should be fired. You are one segment on Fox News I immediately turn off. (User H, comment on Trump/Wallace interview, July 20, 2020)

The negativity aimed at both interviewers was not necessarily about the poor skills or arrogant demeanor of the interviewer, but the fact that the questions posed by Swan and Wallace showed DT in an unkind light. This notion, in particular with respect to Christopher Wallace and Fox News, was picked up by other commentators in an attempt to point out the supporters' hypocritical approach:

> If you want to see how blindly people follow Trump, watch them drop Fox News, a notorious right wing media outlet, like a rock because they're starting to go against what the President is saying. So, who is really wrong here, the bloviating, narcissistic cult leader, or literally everyone else? (User I, comment on Trump/Wallace interview, July 21, 2020)

The above example shows the strong grip with which DT had captured parts of the audience, that is, anyone deciding to challenge DT's utterances or fact-check his statements could expect the status of persona non grata. With respect to this particular interview by Wallace, the temporary or partial ostracism was also extended to Fox News, which is a known stronghold for conservatives and generally shows DT's actions in a positive light (e.g., Grynbaum, 2021).

Explicitly and Implicitly against Donald Trump

Some commentators quickly pointed out the discordance between what DT was asked about in the interview and what DT decided to speak on and why. Expressions of explicit disappointment regarding the way in which DT carried himself during the interviews point to three distinct but closely connected grievances against DT's utterances within the pandemic context: "When questions are being asked, he doesn't let you finish, doesn't answer what was asked, answers to something that wasn't asked, or turns it around to talk about himself . . . " (User J, comment on Trump/Swan interview, August 4, 2020). The above comment takes issue with DT's tendency to twist questions and talking points to shift the conversation towards his own persona.

Here, it is important to note that the decision to resume regular public pandemic briefings with DT in participation immediately followed the Chris Wallace interview on Fox News. In fact, the comments pertaining to the substance of and the reasons for DT's appearances clearly show a disconnect between what some audience members seem to have expected from the interviews, that is, new and accurate information, and what DT delivered in his responses to interview questions. Where DT gave a more or less direct response to the questions put to him, the audience expressed dissatisfaction regarding the substance and veracity of DT's responses: "When has Trump ever had an honest conversation? Also, like Palin, a basic question or questions with facts is a 'gotcha' question for him. Facts don't lie, Trump lies" (User K, comment on Trump/Swan interview, August 4, 2020).

The above also includes a challenge to DT's preparedness for the interview appearances, particularly regarding the Axios on HBO interview in which DT had a difficult time when trying to explain different statistical charts to Jonathan Swan. The account of DT's administration during the COVID-19 pandemic in a book published by the *Washington Post* journalists Abutaleb and Paletta (2021) suggests that the charts were also new to DT. The tendency of DT to make conversations about himself regardless of the topic under discussion or the context within which the conversation takes place was captured as follows:

> He is faultless, he is the truth, if you love him, you're a person of worth, if not, you're worthless. America doesn't have President or a king, it has a wannabe god. (User L, comment on Trump/Swan interview, August 4, 2020)
>
> Ego ego ego . . . What people are dying??? But have you seen how much likes I get?? Did you read about all the fake news they say about me??? Let me explain how great of a guy I am as you ask me about people dying how to save them. (User M, comment on Trump/Swan interview, August 5, 2020)
>
> Trump largely left it up to the states to handle the virus, and that failed miserably. By taking a hands-off approach, he thought he could dust his hands of the problem and absolve himself of any blame. [. . .] You are lying to yourself by saying he never departed from the opinions of experts. He failed to show leadership in this crisis, and we are paying for it. (User N, comment on Trump/Swan interview, August 5, 2020)

The third example brings in the notion of accountability, suggesting that DT had failed to uphold his leadership responsibilities during the pandemic. The wording of the comment shows that it was addressed to a previous commentator, that is, it was an attempt at convincing another viewer that things are not as DT makes them out to be. In general, the comment is characteristic of the sentiment exhibited by audience members explicitly or implicitly against DT. Audience members, who took issue with DT's lack of action during the pandemic, were also the ones to specifically direct attention to the dire reality that, for the most part, only featured as the background aura for the media spectacle:

> Please, somebody, ask directly why he thinks ratings matter. I think I know, but I'd like to hear his (likely rambling) response. For example:
>
> Trump: "We had great ratings, like never before (yada-yada-yada)."
>
> Reporter: "Why are ratings so important to you? You're the President, not a television personality anymore. Ratings are not an appropriate metric of success for anything you do. Why do you keep dwelling on ratings?" (User O, comment on Trump/Swan interview, August 4, 2020)

The above comment is not only a critical assessment of DT's actions (or lack thereof) but is concurrently something that the media establishment ought to be willing to answer about their choices regarding emotionally charged media coverage of DT and the continued fascination with creating a spectacle, i.e., engaging in scandalization practices.

Just Here for the (Dark) Entertainment

Although comments coded as "mockery" could, in principle, have been divided between the for-and-against DT categories, it would have resulted in the loss of an important insight about media coverage of DT's version of crisis communication. This insight concerns the notion of entertainment value sourced from the interviews:

> [. . .] Saved my best weed for this! I knew this would end up turning juicy! I was not disappointed. (User P, comment on Trump/Wallace interview, July 20, 2020)
>
> Great interview, Donnie! Glad you were able to clearly articulate and showcase your plans for Making America Great Again! Sincerely, the Biden campaign. (User Q, comment on Trump/Swan interview, August 4, 2020)
>
> Bahahahaha!!! Trump got rekt! I honestly can't believe people think he is a smart guy. I cried laughing at this interview. (User R, comment on Trump/Wallace interview, July 20, 2020)
>
> That was a great sketch! Who's playing Trump? Awesome acting and they really nailed the make-up. I also love it when the actors have a hard time keeping a straight face, almost breaking the fourth wall . . . adds a bit of warmth to it. What's that? It's a real interview of a guy with access to nukes? I'll be in the

basement, eating beef from a tin. . . . (User S, comment on Trump/Swan interview, August 5, 2020)

The above examples express sarcasm, *schadenfreude*, and an expectation of being entertained. Here, it is important to remember that DT's appearances in the interviews were part of re-establishing DT's presence within the U.S. pandemic-response narrative. The disbelief and sarcasm may be discounted as off-the-cuff reactions based on an already negative attitude towards DT. However, the mockery and sarcasm directed towards DT, or exchanged between supporters and detractors, were so pervasive in the sample (244 of 800 comments) that it necessitated separate attention. The notion of a distinct expectation of being entertained was the most alarming aspect in the findings, given that the interviews were announced as sources of information about a deadly pandemic delivered as a conversation between expert interviewers and the President. Moreover, if audience members had formed an expectation of entertainment, then the media outlets organizing the interviews must have also been aware of the possibility of a spectacle. Based on audience responses, this applies to the Fox News interview even more so than the Axios interview on HBO, which provided that DT's supporters were not expecting to see DT fact-checked during the interview and reacted by accusing the interviewer of being biased and condescending.

There were also those who implicitly questioned the necessity of the interviews in general, for example: "This feels like a spoof interview or something . . . mainly because Trump is a joker who just says the most random things, but the interviewer is pretty comedic (in a good direct way)" (User T, comment on Trump/Swan interview, August 4, 2020). This notion further enforces the possibility that many in the audience were not viewing the interviews to receive pandemic updates and were primarily present for the entertainment that is likely to ensue when DT is placed in front of a camera and, as a commentator sarcastically remarked, asked so-called gotcha questions.

To summarize the audience responses elaborated in more detail above: approximately a third of the reactions were "mockery" either directed at DT or exchanged between supporters and detractors of DT. A further third were "neutral" comments, which mainly addressed the interviewer's actions, and consequently, revealed implicit support or opposition towards DT. The remaining comments were an almost even split along expected and historically well-established partisan lines. Given that the two analyzed interviews were instances of crisis communication, audience reactions to something new being revealed in terms of information were essentially absent from the sample of comments. The audience members were reacting to the persona of DT or aspects relating to the persona of DT, for example, views of supporters, detractors, or the actions of those engaging with DT, and not the novelty of information provided in the interviews.

DISCUSSION

According to Fairbanks, Plowman, and Rawlins (2007), "a healthy democracy requires an informed public and demands that governments provide information to the public about policies, decisions, and actions" (p. 24). Thus, meaningful communication between the government and the public is not merely a managerial practicality but an obligation originating "from the basic covenant between government and the people" (Viteritti, 1997, p. 82, as cited in Liu & Horsley, 2007). This necessity only gets amplified in times of a crisis (Hansson et al., 2020; Kim & Kreps, 2020). Furthermore, the public often interprets government communication as a reflection of how much the government values the public good (Lee, 2009, p. 74). Hence, communication that is truthful and timely, avoids speculation, and connects with the audience (Covello, 2003; Reynolds & Quinn, 2008) must be at the heart of government communication during times of crisis. Based on the audience responses analyzed in the previous section, government risk and crisis communication may not be the most suitable framework for thinking about and analyzing DT's public appearances and communicative choices during the COVID-19 pandemic.

Throughout his presidency, and often in a particularly dramatic manner, DT cast himself as a long-suffering, tormented victim (Leonnig & Rucker, 2021). Put differently, DT operated as a publicly elected character with a backstory, pet peeves, nemeses, ambitions driven by self-interest, and an aura facilitated by self-aggrandizement. This ensemble of characteristics also made him particularly unsuitable for a leadership position in a crisis situation, where public good must be maintained as the focus. As Covello (2003) suggested, health risk and crisis communication ought to be frank and truthful, while avoiding speculation and over-assuring. For DT, providing accurate information would have meant recognizing the many shortcomings in crisis management that occurred under his administration, and not just during the COVID-19 pandemic (see Leonnig & Rucker, 2021). Thus, instead of using transparent government communication as a policy tool (see Howlett, 2009), DT's public appearances became a misinformation-filled and scandal-proposing promotional tool for the main character of the so-called *Trump Show*.

Not only were DT's communications in the two interviews in stark contrast with the recommendations by Covello (2003), but the utterances, and the narrative, were based on the persona of DT (Holpuch, 2020; Schwartz, 2020) rather than the needs of a population in crisis. This was promptly reflected in the more intense (and, at times, visceral) audience's responses, even if not always explicitly. With respect to responses that were likely to be sincere expressions of support, the audience was not reacting to the content of DT's utterances but the fact that it was DT making the statements. Responses that expressed opposition towards DT included disbelief, disappointment, and exhaustion. However, the exhaustion reflected an acknowledgement that the situation under scrutiny has played out in a similar fashion before, and given the opportunity that will likely do so again. In other words, members of the audience who expressed an attitude of disapproval towards DT were tuning in to the interviews only to be disappointed by the carried narrative and the lack of changes or evolution in the cast of characters of the *Trump Show*.

The audience was also split between those who took DT's words as the gold standard that requires no further verification and those who had ceased to believe a single word DT utters. The vitriol created from the split in sentiment was clearly on display in the findings regarding DT and even carried over to assessments of the interviewers. In essence, DT and the interviewer presented as the protagonist and the antagonist—positions that switched depending on the perspective—in an episode of the *Trump Show*. Furthermore, the visceral reactions to the perceived slights of the interviewers suggest that audience members whose attitudes towards DT was supportive viewed the suggested poor treatment of DT as an attempt to kill off the main character of their favorite show. On the other hand, those with a negative attitude towards DT could not wait for the character to be replaced with someone more suitable. The audience, thus, comprised fans and anti-fans (see Gray, 2003) of the *Trump Show*. Considering the relative absence of DT from the public eye following the disinfectant debacle, the fans of the *Trump Show* were present to cast their vote of support. The anti-fans were present in equal numbers to both express their frustrations and restate the various ways in which they considered the *Trump Show* to be "inane, stupid, morally bankrupt and/or aesthetic drivel" (Gray, 2003, p. 70).

The choice of viewing the above as a distinction between fans and anti-fans of the *Trump Show* rather than a disagreement between the supporters and detractors of a particular President is further enforced because DT's pandemic information was not considered particularly trustworthy to begin with (Quinnipiac University, 2020). Ultimately, if new information is not what viewers left with (or came for) but viewership numbers remain consistently high, then some other value must be drawing the crowd. This value is better understood as entertainment value (Dobni, 2007), which is, given the context of a deadly pandemic, sourced from an instance of dark entertainment. For the fans, it was a glimpse of their favorite hero. For the anti-fans, it was an expectation of a "car-crash" (Bump, 2020, para. 17), that is, a promise of *schadenfreude*-based entertainment (see Kuipers, 2014). In retrospect, this expectation was perhaps best captured by the fact that when DT himself contracted COVID-19 in early fall 2020 (O'Key, 2020), searches for the word *schadenfreude* spiked 30,500 percent, according to Merriam-Webster (Foreman, 2020). Where someone becoming infected with a potentially lethal virus is viewed, or at least considered, by others from the perspective of perceived deservingness (Feather, 2014; Powell, 2014), the prior actions or behavior of the infected person must have also been viewed as severe transgressions. The galvanizing effects of DT's pandemic narrative spread across both aisles, inspiring fans and infuriating anti-fans. Thus, while high viewership ratings do not always entail supporting viewers, the consistency in ratings themselves cannot be ignored. Nevertheless, the dark entertainment derived from the *Trump Show* is akin to ignoring or suppressing the fact of a burning apartment building just to laugh at one's neighbors or landlord. In this scenario, the media's current role seems to be to ensure the buildings are well-stocked with gasoline-soaked rags to not waste any potential sparks.

Each individual episode of the *Trump Show* embeds the potential to "go viral" (Peters et al., 2021), that is, to be spread and replicated with enormous speed in the modern information ecosystem (e.g., Yang et al., 2021). Nahon and Hemsley (2013) point out that the virality of information is not new, but the modern information ecosystem enabled an important aspect of virality, that is, the frequency of viral events. Nahon and Hemsley (2013) state that viral content "is what stands out as *remarkable* in a sea of content" (p. 2, the italic emphasis in original). However, when a specific type of character or theme stands out as remarkable in an abundance of content, it ought to lead us to discuss the possibility of *chronic episodes* instead of frequent viral events. DT's obsession with the viewership ratings of his public appearances indicates a wish for the *chronicity* of a subject or topic, i.e., an extended duration for the significance of a topic or person expressed as (ir)regular manifestations or reappearances of said topic or person in viral content. In that sense, the media only played into the desires of DT by providing his coverage in the form of incessant scandalization (see Graβl et al., 2019), regardless of whether DT's particular transgressions were seen as mild or severe. DT as an object of coverage brings high viewership numbers because the chronicity of DT aids in drumming up and maintaining high emotions in a population and media environment split along party lines. The status quo requires a realization that a state opposite to the presence of specific emotions, whether positive or negative, is indifference, not emotions of a different valence. Preston and associates (2021) recently found that emotional intelligence is an important indicator of whether people fall for fake news but also noted that people with lower emotional intelligence might do just as well with non-emotion-based fake news tests. This suggests that the media could, in fact, choose to decrease its own use of emotional appeals when covering controversial sources such as DT.

When viewed from the perspective of audience responses, the idea of chronicity can be used to explain the diverging attitudes expressed towards DT without taking anything away from the apparent popularity of the content itself. Since chronicity requires more than one occurrence, a preceding occurrence drives the subsequent one, which in turn prepares viewers for any number of occurrences that follow. Thus, the regularity with which DT's broadcasted appearances drew noticeable viewership numbers was not about the substance of information disseminated or even the particularities of a crisis but the continued salience of DT in terms of content-based attractiveness to both fans and anti-fans. Hence, the interviews carried out by Christopher Wallace and Jonathan Swan were mere episodes of the *Trump Show*, that is, manifestations of the chronicity of DT. The pandemic narrative of DT was a thin veil for self-promotion in preparation for the (then) upcoming elections. Put differently, the pandemic was yet another pretense for DT to be on television and in full display, for the media to provide incessant emotion-filled coverage of what was essentially a lack of new useful information, and the audience to be inspired or incensed by two new episodes of the dark entertainment that was (and still is) the *Trump Show*.

CONCLUSION

Whether individual instances of mishaps and blunders go "viral" becomes less of an issue if the person depicted has already (long since) become "chronic." In other words, an expectation of entertainment value from the consumption of content featuring DT may already precede individual manifestations of such content. When the purported reasons for the resumption of DT's regular briefings, that is, the importance of getting pandemic information to the American people, are set aside, the objective outcome of DT's appearances based on audience responses to the two interviews analyzed in this chapter were high viewership numbers, strong emotional reactions, and references to being entertained. Outcomes of this nature are eerie reflections of expectations one might have for a popular TV show, not a head of state communicating with the citizens of a country during a deadly pandemic.

Thus, this chapter was able to show that many of the people tuning in for the Fox News and Axios on HBO interviews with DT were not expecting to receive updates about the pandemic—they were expecting another dose of entertainment, that is, fans witnessing their hero take the stage, and anti-fans criticizing a villain that utters lies, uses awkward phrasing, avoids important questions, and tells tall tales about his own role in the pandemic response.

The difficult conclusion is that DT's interviews cannot easily be categorized as crisis communication because the appearances had all the makings of dark entertainment: these were spectacles made possible by a deadly pandemic, powered by partisan divisions among audience members, and capitalized on by an insatiable media apparatus willing to emotionally charge and relentlessly scandalize every manifestation of the chronicity of Donald J. Trump.

NOTES

1. At the time of editing, the original video, from which the comments were collected as data for this chapter, was no longer available for viewing on YouTube. For a working version, see YouTube video "Trump Exclusive Interview Jonathan Swan (Full Interview) AXIOS HBO" (Melmax7, 2020) but the comments are different from those used for the analysis.

REFERENCES

Abutaleb, Y., & Paletta, D. F. (2021). *Nightmare scenario: Inside the Trump administration's response to the pandemic that changed history*. New York: Harper.

Amenabar, T. (2020, September 3). "The 1918 flu is still with us": The deadliest pandemic ever is still causing problems today. *The Washington Post*. Retrieved from https://www.washingtonpost.com/history/2020/09/01/1918-flu-pandemic-end/

Aratani, L. (2020, April 25). Trump says briefings "not worth the effort" amid fallout from disinfectant comments. *The Guardian*. Retrieved from https://www.theguardian.com/us-news/2020/apr/25/donald-trump-stays-away-from-briefings-amid-fallout-from-disinfectant-comments

Axios on HBO. (2020, August 3). *AXIOS on HBO: President Trump exclusive interview (Full Episode) | HBO* [Video]. *YouTube*. Retrieved from https://web.archive.org/web/20200805165839if_/https://www.youtube.com/watch?v=zaaTZkqsaxY

Baker, P., & Haberman, M. (2020, July 20/September 9). After dismissing coronavirus surge, Trump wants to talk about the virus again. *The New York Times*. Retrieved from https://www.nytimes.com/2020/07/20/us/politics/trump-coronavirus-briefings.html

BBC. (2020, April 24). Coronavirus: Outcry after Trump suggests injecting disinfectant as treatment. *BBC*. Retrieved from https://www.bbc.com/news/world-us-canada-52407177

Bond, P. (2016, February 29). Leslie Moonves on Donald Trump: "It may not be good for America, but it's damn good for CBS." *The Hollywood Reporter*. Retrieved from https://www.hollywoodreporter.com/news/general-news/leslie-moonves-donald-trump-may-871464/

Brants, K. (1998). Who's afraid of infotainment? *European Journal of Communication, 13*(3), 315–335. Retrieved from https://doi.org/10.1177/0267323198013003002

Bump, P. (2020, July 20). When Trump was holding regular briefings, his approval was higher. It wasn't because of the briefings. *The Washington Post*. Retrieved from https://www.washingtonpost.com/politics/2020/07/20/when-trump-was-holding-regular-briefings-his-approval-was-higher-it-wasnt-because-briefings/

Clissold, B. (2004). *Candid Camera* and the origins of reality TV: Contextualizing a historical precedent. In S. Holmes & D. Jermyn (Eds.), *Understanding reality television* (pp. 33–53). Routledge.

Covello, V. T. (2003). Best practices in public health risk and crisis communication. *Journal of Health Communication*, *8*(sup. 1), 5–8. Retrieved from https://doi.org/10.1080/713851971

Dobni, D. (2007). Entertainment value: The concept and its dimensions. *Journal of Hospitality & Leisure Marketing*, *15*(4), 5–23. Retrieved from https://doi.org/10.1300/J150v15n04_02

Engell, L. (2005). Fall und fälle: Kleine philosophie des fernsehsskandals [Traps and types: A small philosophy of the television scandal]. In S. Borg, C. Gerhards, & B. Lambert (Eds.), *TV-skandale* (pp. 18–37). Konstanz: UVK.

Fairbanks, J., Plowman, K. D., & Rawlins, B. L. (2007). Transparency in government communication. *Journal of Public Affairs*, *7*, 23–37. Retrieved from https://doi.org/10.1002/pa.245

Feather, N. T. (2014). Deservingness and schadenfreude. In W. W. van Dijk & J. W. Ouwerkerk (Eds.), *Schadenfreude: Understanding pleasure at the misfortune of others* (pp. 29–57). Cambridge, UK: Cambridge University Press.

Feinberg, A. (2020, April 7). Trump is the star of the coronavirus show, and he's loving every minute of it: Who needs rallies? *Slate*. Retrieved from https://slate.com/news-and-politics/2020/04/trump-star-coronavirus-show-press-briefing.html

Foreman, A. (2020, October 3). Merriam-Webster sees 30,500% spike in "schadenfreude" searches following Trump diagnosis. *Mashable*. Retrieved from https://mashable.com/article/dictionary-spike-schadenfreude-trump-coronavirus

Fox News. (2020a, July 19). *President Trump goes one-on-one with Chris Wallace | Full Interview* [Video]. *YouTube*. Retrieved from https://www.youtube.com/watch?v=W6XdpDOH1JA&t=1s&ab_channel=FoxNews

Fox News. (2020b, July 19). Transcript: "Fox News Sunday" interview with President Trump. *Foxnews.com*. Retrieved from https://www.foxnews.com/politics/transcript-fox-news-sunday-interview-with-president-trump

Geiβ, S. (2017). Scandalization. In P. Rössler, C. A. Hoffner, & L. Zoonen (Eds.), *The international encyclopedia of media effects*. *Wiley Online Library*. Retrieved from https://doi.org/10.1002/9781118783764.wbieme0198

Graβl, P., Schaap, G., Spagnuolo, F., & Van't Riet, J. (2019). The effects of scandalization in political news messages on political trust and message evaluation. *Journalism, 22*(10), 2566–2582. Retrieved from https://doi.org/10.1177/1464884919879582

Gray, J. (2003). New audiences, new textualities: Anti-fans and non-fans. *International Journal of Cultural Studies*, *6*(1), 64–81. Retrieved from https://doi.org/10.1177/1367877903006001004

Goldfinch, S., Taplin, R., & Gauld, R. (2021). Trust in government increased during the Covid-19 pandemic in Australia and New Zealand. *Australian Journal of Public Administration, 80*(1), 3–11. Retrieved from https://doi.org/10.1111/1467-8500.12459

Grynbaum, M. M. (2016, December 1). CNN's coverage of Trump was biased, presidential candidates' aides say. *The New York Times*. Retrieved from https://www.nytimes.com/2016/12/01/business/media/trump-cnns-coverage-biased-presidential-candidates-aides-say.html

Grynbaum, M. M. (2020, March 25/July 20). Trump's briefings are a ratings hit. Should networks cover them live? *The New York Times*. Retrieved from https://www.nytimes.com/2020/03/25/business/media/trump-coronavirus-briefings-ratings.html

Grynbaum, M. M. (2021, May 28). Fox News intensifies its pro-Trump politics as dissenters depart. *The New York Times*. Retrieved from https://www.nytimes.com/2021/05/28/business/media/trump-fox-news.html

Guttman, A. (1998). The appeal of violent sports. In J. Goldstein (Ed.), *Why we watch: The attraction of violent entertainment* (pp. 7–26). New York: Oxford University Press.

Hall, S. (1973). Encoding and decoding in television discourse. [Discussion Paper]. University of Birmingham. Retrieved from http://epapers.bham.ac.uk/2962/1/Hall%2C_1973%2C_Encoding_and_Decoding_in_the_Television_Discourse.pdf

Halsey, A., III. (2018, February 3). A killer flu was raging. But in 1918, U.S. officials ignored the crisis to fight a war. *The Washington Post*. Retrieved from https://www.washingtonpost.com/news/retropolis/wp/2018/02/03/a-killer-flu-was-raging-but-in-1918-u-s-officials-ignored-the-crisis-to-fight-a-war/

Hansson, S., Orru, K., Siibak, A., Bäck, A., Krüger, F., Gabel, F., & Morsut, C. (2020). Communication-related vulnerability to disasters: A heuristic framework. *International Journal of Disaster Risk Reduction, 51*, 101931. Retrieved from https://doi.org/10.1016/j.ijdrr.2020.101931

Hansson, S., Orru, K., Torpan, S., Bäck, A., Kazemekaityte, A., Meyer, S. F., Ludvigsen, J., Savadori, L., Galvagni, A., & Pigrée, A. (2021). COVID-19 information disorder: Six types of harmful information during the pandemic in Europe. *Journal of Risk Research, 24*(3–4), 380–393. Retrieved from https://doi.org/10.1080/13669877.2020.1871058

Holpuch, A. (2020, July 20). Donald Trump v Fox News Sunday: Extraordinary moments from a wild interview. *The Guardian*. Retrieved from https://www.theguardian.com/us-news/2020/jul/19/donald-trump-fox-news-sunday-chris-wallace-interview

Howlett, M. (2009). Government communication as a policy tool: A framework for analysis. *The Canadian Political Science Review, 3*(2), 23–37. Retrieved from https://ojs.unbc.ca/index.php/cpsr/article/view/134/184

Hutto, C. J., & Gilbert, E. (2014). VADER: A parsimonious rule-based model for sentiment analysis of social media text. *Proceedings of the Eighth International AAAI Conference on Weblogs and Social Media* (ICWSM, Ann Arbor, Michigan, USA,

June 1–4, 2014), 216–225. The AAAI Press. Retrieved from https://www.aaai.org/ocs/index.php/ICWSM/ICWSM14/paper/view/8109/8122

Jensen, M. (2018). Russian trolls and fake news: Information or identity logics? *Journal of International Affairs, 71*, 115–124. Retrieved from https://www.jstor.org/stable/26508125

Jordan, E. O. (1927). *Epidemic influenza: A survey*. Chicago: University of Chicago Press.

Kendzior, S. (2020). *Hiding in plain sight: The invention of Donald Trump and the erosion of America*. New York: Flatiron Books.

Kessler, G., Rizzo, S., & Kelly, M. (2020). *Donald Trump and his assault on truth: The President's falsehoods, misleading claims and flat-out lies*. New York: Scribner.

Kikerpill, K., & Siibak, A. (2021). Abusing the COVID-19 pan(dem)ic. In J. C. Pollock & D. A. Vakoch (Eds.), *COVID-19 in international media: Global pandemic perspectives* (pp. 249–258). London; New York: Routledge.

Kim, D. K. D., & Kreps, G. L. (2020). An analysis of government communication in the United States during the COVID-19 pandemic: Recommendations for effective government health risk communication. *World Medical & Health Policy, 12*(4), 398–412. Retrieved from https://doi.org/10.1002/wmh3.363

Kuckartz, U. (2019). Qualitative text analysis: A systematic approach. In G. Kaiser & N. Presmeg (Eds.), *Compendium for early career researchers in mathematics education. ICME-13 Monographs* (pp. 181–197). Cham, Switzerland: Springer. Retrieved from https://doi.org/10.1007/978-3-030-15636-7_8

Kuipers, G. (2014). Schadenfreude and social life: A comparative perspective on the expression and regulation of mirth at the expense of others. In W. W. van Dijk & J. W. Ouwerkerk (Eds.), *Schadenfreude: Understanding pleasure at the misfortune of others* (pp. 259–274). Cambridge, UK: Cambridge University Press.

Lee, K. (2009). How the Hong Kong government lost the public trust in SARS: Insights for government communication in a health crisis. *Public Relations Review, 35*(1), 74–76. Retrieved from https://doi.org/10.1016/j.pubrev.2008.06.003

Leonnig, C., & Rucker, P. (2021). *I alone can fix it: Donald J. Trump's catastrophic final year*. New York: Penguin Press.

Liptak, K. (2020, July 21). Trump says briefings will return and touts masks, in apparent shift amid surge in Covid cases. *CNN Politics*. Retrieved from https://edition.cnn.com/2020/07/20/politics/donald-trump-coronavirus-briefings/index.html

Liu, B. F., & Horsley, J. S. (2007). The government communication decision wheel: Toward a public relations model for the public sector. *Journal of Public Relations Research, 19*(4), 377–393. Retrieved from https://doi.org/10.1080/10627260701402473

Liu, B. F., Iles, I. A., & Herovic, E. (2020). Leadership under fire: How governments manage crisis communication. *Communication Studies, 71*(1), 128–147. Retrieved from https://doi.org/10.1080/10510974.2019.1683593

Mason, L. (2018). *Uncivil agreement: How politics became our identity*. Chicago: University of Chicago Press.

Melmax7. (2020, August 8). Trump exclusive interview Jonathan Swan (Full Interview) *AXIOS HBO* [Video, original date on July 28, 2020]. *YouTube*.

Retrieved from https://www.youtube.com/watch?v=yJIhxKFH9gI&t=4s&ab_channel=melmax7

Miller, L. J. (2019). Feelings trump facts: Affect and the rhetoric of Donald Trump. In L. Zhang & C. Clark (Eds.), *Affect, emotion, and rhetorical persuasion in mass communication* (pp. 195–204). New York: Routledge.

Miroff, B. (2018). The presidential spectacle. In M. Nelson (11th ed.), *The presidency and the political system* (pp. 257–279). Thousand Oaks, CA: SAGE/CQ Press.

Mizrahi, S., Vigoda-Gadot, E., & Cohen, N. (2021). How well do they manage a crisis? The government's effectiveness during the COVID-19 pandemic. *Public Administration Review*. *Wiley Online Library*. Retrieved from https://doi.org/10.1111/puar.13370

Morens, D. M., Taubenberger, J. K., & Fauci, A. S. (2021). A centenary tale of two pandemics: The 1918 influenza pandemic and COVID-19, Part I. *American Journal of Public Health*, *111*(6), 1086–1094. Retrieved from https://doi.org/10.2105/AJPH.2021.306310

Nahon, K., & Hemsley, J. (2013). *Going viral*. Cambridge, UK: Polity.

Ogbodo, J. N., Onwe, E. C., Chukwu, J., Nwasum, C. J., Nwakpu, E. S., Nwankwo, S. U., Nwamini, S., Elem, S., & Ogbaeja, N. I. (2020). Communicating health crisis: A content analysis of global media framing of COVID-19. *Health Promotion Perspectives*, *10*(3), 257–269. Retrieved from https://doi.org/10.34172/hpp.2020.40

O'Key, S. (2020, October 12). A timeline of Trump's battle with Covid-19. [Photo Editors: Tuazon, B., Roegiers, B., Lanzoni, W., & Almond, K.]. *CNN*. Retrieved from https://edition.cnn.com/interactive/2020/10/politics/trump-covid-battle/

Peters, M. A., McLaren, P., & Jandrić, P. (2021). A viral theory of post-truth. *Educational Philosophy and Theory*. *Taylor & Francis Online*. Retrieved from https://doi.org/10.1080/00131857.2020.1750090

Peters, J. W., Plott, E., & Haberman, M. (2020, April 26). 260,000 words, full of self-praise, from Trump on the virus. *The New York Times*. Retrieved from https://www.nytimes.com/interactive/2020/04/26/us/politics/trump-coronavirus-briefings-analyzed.html

Posner, R. A. (1995). *Overcoming law*. Cambridge, MA: Harvard University Press.

Powell, C. A. J. (2014). Hypocrisy and schadenfreude. In W. W. van Dijk & J. W. Ouwerkerk (Eds.), *Schadenfreude: Understanding pleasure at the misfortune of others* (pp. 58–74). Cambridge, UK: Cambridge University Press.

Preston, S., Anderson, A., Robertson, D. J., Shephard, M. P., & Huhe, N. (2021). Detecting fake news on Facebook: The role of emotional intelligence. *PLOS ONE*, *16*(3), e0246757. Retrieved from https://doi.org/10.1371/journal.pone.0246757

Quinnipiac University. (2020, July 15). Biden widens lead over Trump to 15 points in presidential race, Quinnipiac University national poll finds; Trump job approval rating drops to 36 percent. *Quinnipiac University*. Retrieved from https://poll.qu.edu/Poll-Release?releaseid=3781

Rev. (2020, August 3). Donald Trump interview transcript with Jonathan Swan of Axios on HBO [Video, Transcript]. *REV.com*. Retrieved from https://www.rev.com/blog/transcripts/donald-trump-interview-transcript-with-axios-on-hbo

Reynolds, B., & Quinn, S. C. (2008). Effective communication during an influenza pandemic: The value of using a crisis and emergency risk communication framework. *Health Promotion Practice*, *9* (sup. 4), 13S–17S. doi: 10.1177/1524839908325267

Sample, C., Jensen, M. J., Scott, K., McAlaney, J., Fitchpatrick, S., Brockinton, A., Ormrod, D., & Ormrod, A. (2020). Interdisciplinary lessons learned while researching fake news. *Frontiers in Psychology*, *11*, 537612. doi: 10.3389/fpsyg.2020.537612

Sayre, S., & King, C. (2003). *Entertainment and society: Audiences, trends and impact*. Thousand Oaks, CA: SAGE Publications, Inc.

Schreier, M. (2014). Qualitative content analysis. In U. Flick (Ed.), *The SAGE handbook of qualitative data analysis* (pp. 170–183). Thousand Oaks, CA: SAGE Publications, Inc.

Schwartz, M. (2020, August 19). The Axios interview showed us an important threshold for the president. *The New York Times Magazine*. Retrieved from https://www.nytimes.com/2020/08/19/magazine/trump-axios-interview.html

Seeger, M. W., Sellnow, T. L., & Ulmer, R. R. (2003). *Communication and organizational crisis*. Westport, CT: Praeger.

Sheppard, S. I. (2008). *The partisan press: A history of media bias in the United States*. Jefferson, NC: McFarland & Co.

Stahl, M. (2018, October 2). Subversion gone wrong: Inside "bumfights." *Rolling Stone*. Retrieved from https://www.rollingstone.com/culture/culture-features/bumfights-homeless-men-fight-activists-730393/

Tomes, N. (2010). "Destroyer and Teacher": Managing the masses during the 1918–1919 influenza pandemic. *Public Health Reports*, *125*(Sup. 3), 48–62. Retrieved from https://doi.org/10.1177/00333549101250S308

Tsipursky, G. (2017, February 21). Towards a post-lies future: Fighting "alternative facts" and "post-truth" politics. *The Humanist*. Retrieved from https://thehumanist.com/magazine/march-april-2017/features/towards-post-lies-future/

Viteritti, J. P. (1997). The environmental context of communication: Public sector organizations. In J. L. Garnett & A. Kouzmin (Eds.), *Handbook of administrative communication* (pp. 79–100). New York: Marcel Dekker.

Vorberg, L., & Zeitler, A. (2019). "This is (not) entertainment!": Media constructions of political scandal discourses in the 2016 US presidential election. *Media, Culture & Society*, *41*(4), 417–432. Retrieved from https://doi.org/10.1177/0163443719833288

World Health Organization. (2020, September 23). Managing the COVID-19 infodemic: Promoting healthy behaviours and mitigating the harm from misinformation and disinformation. Retrieved from https://www.who.int/news/item/23-09-2020-managing-the-covid-19-infodemic-promoting-healthy-behaviours-and-mitigating-the-harm-from-misinformation-and-disinformation

Worldometer. (2021, July 30). COVID-19 coronavirus pandemic. *Worldometers.info* [Data updated daily]. Retrieved from https://www.worldometers.info/coronavirus/#countries

Yang, K.-C., Pierri, F., Hui, P.-M., Axelrod, D., Torres-Lugo, C., Bryden, J., & Menczer, F. (2021). The COVID-19 infodemic: Twitter versus Facebook. *Big Data*

& Society [The special theme issue on "Studying the COVID-19 Infodemic at Scale"], (May), 1–16. Retrieved from https://doi.org/10.1177/20539517211013861

Zaharna, R. S. (2018). *New realities in foreign affairs: Diplomacy in the 21st century.* Berlin: German Institute for International and Security Affairs.

Zuckerman, E. (2020, August 7). The amazing disappearing election. *The Atlantic*. Retrieved from https://www.theatlantic.com/politics/archive/2020/08/why-news-sounds-same/615070/

Chapter Eight

Manufacturing Disinformation

The Story of Plandemic

Stephen D. Caldes, Zach Justus,
and Jennifer A. Malkowski

When COVID-19 emerged rather suddenly onto the scene, the current media ecology provided new, rich access points for conspiratorial theorizing regarding all elements of the virus. Conspiracies have a well-established history, but the marriage of social media and digital storytelling has changed just how pervasive and infective they are, resulting in new threats to public knowledge, democracy, and civil society (Merlan, 2019). Scholars from across disciplines continue to track and examine conspiracies to better understand and theorize the appeal and influence (Rosenblum & Muirhead, 2019). The exponential increase of conspiracy theories in times of crisis is nothing new. Both the Black Death and the 1918 Spanish flu created a significant rise in conspiracy theories (Dacombe, 2021), as did September 11th (Graff, 2020) and recent U.S. mass shooting events (Siemaszko, 2017). Where there is tragedy and confusion, there is often a void; where there is a void, there are slapdash attempts to fill it.

In spring 2020, much of the world lived in an ever-growing void as vetted information and scientific facts about COVID-19 were still in the nascent stages. On April 29, 2020, Ed Yong, science writer for the *Atlantic,* noted that much about the pandemic was still "maddeningly unclear" (para. 3). To wear a mask or not? Disinfect groceries or don't? Quarantine or conduct business as usual? We were a world confused and in crisis. Yong (2020) attributed this confusion to both the scale and pace of the pandemic—quicker and broader than any of recent history—but ultimately concluded that the pandemic was a "problem . . . too big for any one person to fully comprehend" (para. 5). And while U.S. public health officials worked to communicate what they knew, competing theories and misinformation began to trickle in at first, then gush.

Five days after Yong's comments, the video *Plandemic: The Hidden Agenda Behind Covid-19* was released online[1] (Willis, 2020a). In less than the span of twenty-six minutes, the documentary-style video "weaves a grand conspiracy theory by using a host of false and misleading claims about the novel coronavirus pandemic and its origins, vaccines, treatments for COVID-19, and more" (Fichera et al., 2020, para. 2). The video elicited strong mainstream reactions as many popular medical professionals, fact-checking organizations, and social media personalities conducted extensive investigations into the film's claims alongside journalism industry stalwarts (see, for example, Neuman, 2020). Outlandish assertions made in the video, like masks can "activate" COVID-19 (Willis, 2021a, 20:29) and ventilators can "kill" COVID-19 patients (Willis, 2021a, 15:18) were painstakingly debunked (Enserink & Cohen, 2020; Pappas 2020). Within weeks the "viral conspiracy theory video" was removed and denounced across most mainstream social media sites, but not before reaching millions of viewers (Andrews, 2020, para. 1).

Although the viral video's "information" has been debunked and its "main character" discredited, *Plandemic* and the principles within continue to surface, circulate, and influence the status of COVID-19 conversations, even among audiences outside of the conspiracy community. Evidence of the long-lasting impact of the video is plentiful. Willis landed a book deal (Willis, 2021b), Dr. Mikovits has developed a rabid and broad fan base (Dickson, 2020), and the U.S. continues to have a lethally low level of vaccination attributed to disinformation-born hesitancy (Islam et al., 2021). In December 2020, a poll by the Kaiser Family Foundation found that 29 percent of respondents were hesitant about the vaccines, which could significantly impair our ability to reach herd immunity (Hamel, Kirzinger, Muñana, & Brodie, 2020). Earlier that same year, a Pew Research Center study identified *Plandemic* as a notably effective catalyst for sowing seeds of doubt (Mitchell, Jurkowitz, Oliphant, & Shearer, 2020). Even disproven, *Plandemic*'s consequences persist. This chapter unpacks this ongoing public health conundrum by investigating the persuasive tactics at work in *Plandemic*. In doing so, we theorize the dynamic power of merging digital storytelling with narrative nonfiction to manufacture disinformation in/for our contemporary media ecology.

THE STORY OF *PLANDEMIC*

Directed and narrated by Mikki Willis, a self-proclaimed "father/filmaker" [sic] (Willis, 2021a, 00:59), *Plandemic* was self-released on YouTube in early

May 2020. The video is organized around the testimonial interview of discredited virologist Dr. Judy Mikovits (Esnerink & Cohen, 2020), who presents herself as a whistleblower exposing a vast conspiracy of public manipulation involving key figures in response to COVID-19, including Dr. Anthony Fauci (Director of the U.S. National Institute of Allergy and Infectious Diseases), Dr. Robert Redfield (former Director of the Centers for Disease Control and Prevention), and Bill Gates (American software developer, investor, author, and philanthropist). *Plandemic*'s audience is anyone who does not want to be made a fool, and its thrust is that people are dying, economies are folding, and a doomsday is on the horizon, all because an elite few want more money, more fame, and more power. While this thesis could be considered amateurish, it is possible that the veteran narrative moves *Plandemic* makes, and its overall familiar, professional appearance, are exactly what led to its virality.

Adherents of the QAnon conspiracy theory supercharged the spread of the video across the internet, and it quickly went, for lack of a better term, viral, dwarfing other digital fodder from the same time, before ultimately becoming a "mainstream phenomenon" (Frenkel, Decker, & Alba, 2020, para. 10). Within days of its release, it had garnered over 8 million views, nearly unprecedented for a video that cost less than $2,000 to produce (Rottenberg & Perman, 2020). By late spring it was everywhere across multiple platforms, including Facebook, Reddit, YouTube, and Instagram, before it was taken down by mainstream social networks later that year (Brewster, 2020). Reader (2021) writes, "*Plandemic* was the first big wave in a rising tide of unquellable disinformation and misinformation about COVID-19. By the time the internet platforms we rely on to curate the web suppressed the video, it was already too late" (para. 3).

Willis, *Plandemic*'s director, did not originally intend for the roughly twenty-six-minute video to remain a standalone film; he released it as a preview, "teaser," or "first installment" for a forthcoming, full-length documentary (Roose, 2020; Rottenberg & Perman, 2020). That full-length feature, *Plandemic: Indoctrination*, was released on August 18, 2020, but never reached the viewership figures of its predecessor (Newton, 2020b). However, the enthusiasm generated by *Plandemic*'s first installment was enough to land Willis a book deal and dub it to be "the most seen and censored documentary in history" (Willis, 2021b). However dubious the claim, despite being officially banned from numerous popular online platforms (Andrews, 2020), *Plandemic* is still available through Rumble.com and BitChute.com, and enthusiasm for the project has not yet faded on free speech imageboards and right-wing platforms like Parler (Baines, Ittefaq, & Abwao, 2021). This may be because good stories make lasting impressions.

THE POWER OF STORY

An expertly-spun narrative is akin to a narcotic, it envelopes and entrances. The power of story has been noted across time, place, and discipline. Stories are known to shape experiences (Coles, 1989), give human existence meaning (Polkinghorne, 1988), and serve integrally in both knowledge-construction and the shaping of our future (Konnikova, 2015). When defining "man," literary theorist Kenneth Burke (1968) simply reduced him to a "symbol-using . . . animal" (p. 16) and argued that symbols are created solely to use in stories "to give order to human experience and . . . induce others to dwell in them to establish ways of living" (Fisher, 1984, p. 6). Building from Burke's definition, Walter Fisher (1984) later proposed a new "root metaphor" to punctuate and describe the essential nature of human beings: *homo narrans*, which translates to "storytelling human" (p. 6).

At their core, Fisher (1984) understood humans as an employer of story for personal expression, for relating truths about the human condition, and for connecting the lives of "those who have lived, who live now, and who will live in the future" (p. 6). In his landmark essay, "Narration as a Human Communication Paradigm: The Case of Public Moral Argument," Fisher situated storytelling at the center of a newly proposed theory of human communication where *narrative rationality* is essential to navigating both everyday and public life. "In short," according to Fisher (1984), "good reasons are the stuff of stories, the means by which humans realize their nature as reasoning-valuing animals" (p. 8). If human nature relies on story, then a narrative paradigm—a master worldview, be it *fact or fiction*, that orders our world and helps us navigate through it—becomes essential to human existence. In such a paradigm, rationality is dependent upon coherent stories (*narrative probability*) that resonate with our lived experiences (*narrative fidelity*). It may contrast with the dominant "rational world paradigm" that prioritizes logical argument and the scientific method, but Fisher (1984) assures us, that the narrative paradigm is commensurate with that worldview. Moreover, it is useful to/for rational world paradigm enthusiasts. Scientists are humans, after all.

Most (if not all) popular and academic investigations into the persuasive dynamics of *Plandemic* thus far have focused on the "what" is being said in the film. In rhetorical terms, this type of investigation has prioritized understanding and challenging logical appeals at work in the video's explicit message (see, for example, Cook, van der Linden, Lewandowsky, & Ecker, 2020). "Search for [*Plandemic*] now and you'll see a pop-up from an independent fact checker and many videos of doctors debunking its claims" (Newton, 2020a, para. 17). This approach reflects a well-worn response for combating disinformation: public officials and scientists refute, ridicule, and condemn disinformation as "fake news" and then flood the public sphere with "the truth" (a.k.a., a bunch of vetted, scientific information that disproves each problematic claim using tools born from and aligned with a rational world paradigm). However, the ongoing presence of long-debunked conspiracies suggests clear limitations to this *logical, rational* approach. Case in point: there are likely more "flat Earthers" (or, at the very least, flat-earth-curious individuals) alive today than at any other point in history! (Picheta, 2019).

Why, even when we learn information is false—*even when we engage in critical thinking and can spot the outrageous, amateurish, or debunked conspiracy*—why, as consumers of manufactured disinformation, might we depart feeling less sure about what we know and whom to trust? To answer this question, we look closely at specific rhetorical strategies used in *Plandemic* to appeal to the *homo narran* in all of us. Ultimately, *Plandemic* tells a damn good story. And it does so in a fertile media environment that has fundamentally changed how we, as storytelling creatures, navigate truth, life, and tough decisions.

THE *PLANDEMIC* STORY

As author/scholar Maria Konnikova (2015) notes, a well-told narrative helps us "let down our guard" and is ultimately a very "powerful tool of deception" (para. 12). "When a fact is plausible," she continues, "we still need to test it. When a story is plausible, we often assume it's true" (para. 14). In the case of *Plandemic,* we encounter a mixture of information that appears scientific, wrapped in a compelling and cohesive story, offering certainty in a time of frustration and ambiguity, and it is all delivered in a format that feels familiar and true.

Plandemic opens with sepia-toned slow-motion footage of our filmmaker and main character walking, talking, and laughing in a park as a voiceover, borrowing from Freytag's (2004) pyramid of dramatic structure, outlines the *selective* context ("one of the most accomplished scientists of her generation") (Willis, 2021a, 00:14) and the *dire, emotional* exposition ("as the fate of nations hangs in the balance") (Willis, 2021a, 00:49) to create an *us-against-them* conflict ("expose deadly secrets . . . and name names of those behind this plague of corruption that places all human life in danger") (Willis, 2021a, 00:54). With the structure set, the artifice that follows is a masterclass in aping the television news magazine segment a la *60 Minutes*: two makeup'd and mic'd up talking heads float in a well-lit, but unrecognizable void volleying questions and claims as stock photography, B-roll footage, and infographics season the filmed conversation. The interview serves as our baseline as uncontextualized clips of government raids, caution tape,

Fox News, bustling hospitals, random medical bric-a-brac, and screenshots of webpages and academic studies pepper the screen. Nearly the entire video proceeds in this fashion, and in that way, it is strikingly similar to the narrative format for contemporary digital nonfiction. The roles the interviewer and interviewee play are equally as familiar.

Within this interview structure, Dr. Mikovits functions as our subject-narrator, with Willis acting as "reporter"—although a more apt descriptor would be "presenter"—who frequently prompts Dr. Mikovits with questions or cues to move the story along. Mikovits speaks as Willis pulls the levers. She says "a publication last year," he flashes the title page of a scholarly article on the screen (Willis, 2021a, 18:35); when it's insinuated that so many other doctors believe the same thing as her, he fills the screen with a dozen webcammed faces of people wearing scrubs (Willis, 2021a, 13:18); she quotes (without context) a partial clause by White House Coronavirus Response Coordinator Dr. Birx, Willis synchs up the clips and lips seamlessly (Willis, 2021a, 12:50). She is the story; he is the canvas she paints it on.

The story she tells dates back to the early scientific study of HIV/AIDS. As *Plandemic*'s "main character" and our subject-narrator—our guide, the lens/perspective through which we will be presented a claim—her ethos is critical, imperative, and so, from the first lines of the film, there are extensive efforts to write her credibility into the story: "Dr. Judy Mikovits has been called one of the most accomplished scientists of her generation" (Willis, 2021a, 00:14). Additionally, we quickly learn Dr. Mikovits (1) is revered, or at least was, by her colleagues and other medical experts; (2) has exposed a medical truth that the government was trying to hide *before*—and is poised to do it again, even though she knows the consequences intimately; (3) is whistleblowing on this now because she cares not just about our "freedom" as Americans, but for "humanity" in general (Willis, 2021a, 04:02); (4) is *not* some wacky anti-vaxxer; (5) is not a lone wolf, as "so many" other doctors feel similarly (Willis, 2021a, 13:17). When "so many" is uttered, Willis fills the frame with fourteen other doctors/nurses/medical professional/people wearing scrubs—thus creating the spectacle of a large, critical group—but really, it is just *fourteen* other medical professionals of unknown provenance; a drop in the bucket. Regardless, before her tale even begins, she has been shaped as brave, smart, and someone to trust.

Similarly, for us to further believe her story, which is more or less the antithesis of Dr. Anthony Fauci's *story,* work must be done to discredit him. Thus, through rapid and cliché character assassination techniques, Fauci is quickly turned into a villain, someone with *anti-ethos,* someone *incredible, unbelievable, untrustworthy,* a man with a *nefarious "agenda" (*Willis, 2021a, 04:02). He is quickly characterized as a jealous bully hell-bent on fame over the lives of millions of Americans. Early in the video, when the story focuses on 1980s HIV/AIDS research in which Dr. Mikovits took part, it is alleged that Dr. Fauci and others covered up a breakthrough Dr. Mikovits made and, as such, incited the deaths of millions of people. This work dually buttresses her credibility as an insider and sets the stage for the video to attack Dr. Fauci. Willis and Dr. Mikovits bridge the alleged crimes of Dr. Fauci regarding HIV into the current pandemic with this critical exchange:

> Willis: So, Anthony Fauci, the man who is heading the pandemic task force, was involved in a cover-up?
>
> Dr. Mikovits: He directed the cover-up, and in fact everybody else was paid off and paid off big time. Millions of dollars in funding from Tony Fauci, Tony Fauci's organization National Institute of Allergy and Infectious Disease. These investigators that committed the fraud continue to this day to be paid big time by the NIAID.
>
> Willis: And the whole world is listening to his advice to handle this current pandemic. How do we know that what he's saying is what we need to be learning?
>
> Dr. Mikovits: What he's saying is absolute propaganda and the same kind of propaganda he perpetrated to kill millions since 1984. (Willis, 2021a, 04:04–04:54)

This exchange also marks the transition in the video from a focus on past events to the COVID-19 pandemic. However, the character assault on Dr. Fauci continues in the same themes and tones.

In one particular scene, as Dr. Mikovits is talking about how much fame and fortune will fall on Fauci if he convinces everyone a vaccine is required for this virus, we zoom in on a photo of Dr. Fauci with Nancy Pelosi (Democratic Speaker of the House from the 12th Congressional District in California who is despised by much of the far right), Elton John (a flamboyant homosexual who has contributed heavily to Democratic campaigns over the years), and Henry Waxman (a Jewish former Democratic Representative from California) (Willis 2021a, 11:42). The photo is both a dog-whistle for many anti-government far-right conspiracy theorists and the last straw in terms of whom we cannot trust (Fauci) and whom we can (Mikivits). Parched by lies for too long, viewers are now ready for some Kool-Aid.

Further compounding these individual issues of trust was the period of national confusion and frustration with COVID-19 that coincided with the release of *Plandemic*. The inconsistency of state responses in the U.S. was confounded by a mixed federal response sometimes involving direct tension within the task force led by then Vice President Mike Pence. *Plandemic* tells a compelling story of a whistleblower exposing decades of corruption involving many key players and agencies at the center of the COVID-19 response. So, while it is a piece of propaganda and rife with falsehoods, it also allows people who were predisposed to a particular cluster of interpretations to graft those onto their situation. Specifically, *Plandemic* stakes out the ground that masks and lockdowns are bad, Dr. Anthony Fauci is a liar, and that hydroxychloroquine is a widely available wonder drug. At one point, Dr. Mikovits links the suppression of hydroxychloroquine to the delisting of a cheap anti-autism drug she helped to discover and blames it all on major players: "What did Bayer and Monsanto do? They took it away from everybody. You couldn't get it to save your life right now. We tried, believe me, every way we could. So, when you take away a medicine and not just the WHO, the FDA, the CDC, Tony Fauci, close everything" (Willis 2021a, 17:31). So again, we have a historically-based attack on the institutions and key players in the pandemic response combined with allusions to key issues for conspiracists like the connections between the pharmaceutical industry and autism. These ideas could be found in a variety of communities prior to the release of *Plandemic*. Alternative wellness enthusiasts and many conservatives were adamantly opposed to lockdowns and masks (Cheetham, 2021). President Trump himself was a major promoter of hydroxychloroquine (Cathey, 2020), and conservative media had already started to turn on Dr. Fauci (Wilson, 2020). Individually these things are talking points. *Plandemic* animated them into a captivating story complete with history, cover-ups, villains, heroes, fools, and roles to play for everyone, even the audience.

Plandemic provides the viewer with an important storytelling component—a place for themselves. As much a presenter/"reporter," Willis also serves as the stand-in for the critical thinking viewer. He carefully positions himself as a non-believer on a redemption journey throughout the film. Willis presents as open-minded and, at times, even skeptical. He nods along with Dr. Mikovits as she speaks but also often presents a look of deep concern—furrowed brow, squinty-eyed, questioning stare—as if he, too, is learning this information for the first time. He also asks naïve questions as a stand-in for the audience, like "How can a man who's giving global advice for health own a patent in the solution, in the vaccine? Isn't that a conflict of interest, or shouldn't it be?" (Willis 2021a, 08:03). These strawman, nearly rhetorical questions, are part and parcel of the investigative journalism theatre like *Dateline* and the podcast *Serial*. During one pivotal moment, Willis sheepishly queries, "So I have to ask you, are you anti-vaccine?" to which Dr. Mikovits replies, "Oh, absolutely not" (Willis 2021a, 10:04). As the film progresses, Willis mirrors the journey the audience is supposed to be on. He receives some fantastical information, asks questions, and then becomes a true believer. This transition is witnessed in the ways his critical facial expressions soften into smiles, and his hardball journalist cadence shifts to a more conversational tone. As the film concludes, Willis asks how medical professionals should consider their complicity in this tragedy, and Mikovits responds, "forgive yourselves"

(Willis 2021a, 23:30), effectively giving the audience an out for their past transgressions and enlisting them as evangelists for this new truth.

Plandemic is, ultimately, a redemption story, and Willis models what it looks like to be a critical but open and reasonable listener, one that undergoes a conversion in the face of new, compelling information. This does more than provide the audience with a place for themselves; it provides them with another familiar trope. The redemption or conversion story features prominently across genres and consumers of pop culture, but it is especially important for religious consumers. Whether it be Johnny Cash or the Apostle Paul, the stories of redemption contain the same attributes: a flawed character has an important experience, comes to see the truth, and becomes redeemed. In most instances, the newly converted individual now plays a role in evangelizing to others. *Plandemic* shares many of these same attributes, with Dr. Mikovits serving as an outcast prophet and Willis/the viewer serving as the redeemed. For religious, especially evangelical Christian viewers, the story is quite familiar. However, even beyond overt religious similarities, the redemption story is common in popular culture and serves as an easy and welcome point of connection.

Plandemic also follows a popular anti-establishment whistleblower storyline, which is a redemption tale of sorts. The story of an insider blowing the lid off of a corrupt bureaucracy is a shopworn one, to say the least. Even if we primarily are interested in recently produced documentary films, we are still left with more content than we could list. Recent well-received documentaries like *Icarus* (2017), *The Crime of the Century* (2021), and the expansive series *Dirty Money* (2018) all contain common elements of expansive bureaucracies, greedy individuals, a blissfully ignorant public, and corruption that often forces non-elites into exploited status. Many of these even feature extensive healthcare or pharmaceutical elements and all of them feature heroic whistleblowers who have had enough. Superficially, *Plandemic* shares common attributes with many of these well-received documentaries. The story of Dr. Mikovits as an outcast for uncovering the truth is laid out in the first few minutes, and shortly thereafter, her story of persecution as a truth-teller is laid out, including a stint in jail on "no charges" (Willis 2021a, 02:00). The tone for the entire film is then laid out with this exchange: Willis asks, "Apparently their attempt to silence you has failed, and . . . so how do you sit here with confidence to call out these great forces and not fear for your life as you leave this building?" (Willis 2021a, 03:46). Mikovits responds: "Because if we don't stop this now, we can not only forget our Republic and our freedom, but we can forget humanity because we'll be killed by this agenda" (Willis 2021a, 04:02). Within these first minutes of the video, Mikovits, a now established truth-telling outsider who has been ruthlessly persecuted, is nonetheless speaking out because *the stakes are simply too high*. If you watched *Dirty Money* (or *Blackfish* [2013] or *Gasland* [2010] or *The Corporation* [2003] or *The Last Mountain* [2011] or any number of other investigative documentaries hell-bent on exposing the hidden truth), this tone and these plot points feel mighty familiar. Government bureaucrats and pharmaceutical companies are easy targets. The narrative structure and even the characters sound familiar to the viewer. There is no shortage of corruption within government or in the pharmaceutical industry—and these parts of the story sound true because they are true and have been echoed in countless stories and documentaries in the last decade.

PSEUDO-DOCUMENTARY: HOW TO MANUFACTURE DISINFORMATION

While narratives, in general, are highly effective and convincing, digital storytelling has proven to be especially powerful, given that it can look similar to our new favorite way to educate ourselves and stay informed: the documentary. Although the categorization is somewhat controversial among media scholars, filmmakers, and journalists, documentaries can be understood as one form of narrative nonfiction, a form that is now omnipresent in a digital world. From true crime podcasts to "ripped from the headlines" murder and justice documentaries to television news magazines to, maybe especially, the "snackable" digital nano-documentaries we scroll through endlessly on our mobile devices, our appetite for digital nonfiction content is nearly insatiable. If the story is told in the *right way*—that is, a way we know and recognize, a way that feels familiar and, according to Fisher (1984), "ring[s] true" (p. 8)—even if it delivers questionable novelties, incredible coincidences, or logical fallacies, our tendency is to believe it/in it. And *Plandemic* is most definitely presented in this familiar, professional-looking, digital nonfiction form.

In *Plandemic,* we witness savvy rhetorical techniques, ones that rely on the power of a good story, ones that masterfully weave together ethos, pathos, and logos appeals. But even more so, we witness a familiar package, one that capitalizes on recognizable genres to, at most, mobilize conspiracy theorists, and at the very least, introduce uncertainty into a general(ly educated and reasonable) public. *Plandemic* mimics the narrative nonfiction genre—true stories written in the style of fiction novels—so well that even recent, academic, critical investigations into the video refer to it unabashedly as "a documentary" (Nazar & Pieters, 2021, para. 1), a term accurately reserved only for media that provides verifiably factual reports. To be fair, to some extent, all documentaries are potentially dangerous. As media critic Neil Postman (1985) pointed out, truth encased in drama can be a threat to both knowledge in general and democracy in particular. However, slapdash documentaries rife with bias, nefarious purpose (like disinformation campaigns), and myriad debunked facts are, *if they look the part*, magnitudes more hazardous. As Postman noted decades ago in *Amusing Ourselves to Death*, the information itself is secondary to the packaging; "the quality and usefulness of their goods are subordinate to the artifice of their display" (1985, p. 22).

For a long time, the narrative nonfiction genre was mostly disregarded—considered unethical—by both academics and purveyors of *serious* public-facing communication alike; however, over the years, popular and mainstream media outlets seized on its power (for context, see Gutkind, 2006, 2012; Hesse, 2008; Lopate, 2013). From comedy "news" programs to streaming documentaries, entertaining "information" is coming at us faster than ever before. And truthfully, when narrative techniques and imagistic, pathetic appeals are used in ways that bolster quantitative research and substantiate factual/rational evidence, nonfiction can become both less boring (i.e., more engaging) and a very powerful tool for awareness-raising and/or positive change (Caulley, 2008). This marriage—hard facts and powerful storytelling—could be what eventually wakes the nation from its apathy regarding climate change: simply telling us about rising ocean temperatures (fact) without painting a picture of a starving polar bear adrift at sea on an ever-melting wedge of ice (story) is an opportunity missed. However, without a logical backbone and ethical soul, slick and flashy, empty and ominous, nefarious or well-intentioned "nonfiction" narratives such as *Plandemic* can move a people further from the truth, safety, and even freedom. The question now becomes: can a marriage of hard facts (which take time) and powerful storytelling compete with a marriage of conspiracy theory and powerful storytelling?

Communicating effective arguments and factual information to large amounts of people quickly has been a necessity of democratic governments since always, but it is especially the case amidst a global pandemic. But communicating complex information appropriately, proportionally (i.e., raising the *right* amount of fear in people), and understandably (i.e., *jargon-free*) to the general public takes time. Crisis communication is a complex and laborious process with myriad roadblocks and potential landmines (Rakedzon, Segev, Chapnik, Yosef, & Baram-Tsabari, 2017). Even when done well and in line with a rational ethic, public health communication does not always get it right. And when new facts emerge that falsify previous public health messages—which describes early COVID-19 realities where scientific facts often emerged after precautionary advice and mandates were enacted—the status of public health communication as propaganda—biased information that promotes a particular point of view—comes to the fore.

While often considered pejorative, government propaganda is compulsory. Borrowing heavily from Aldous Huxley (1958), Neil Postman, in his 1977 book *Stupid Talk, Crazy Talk*, in an effort to remove the sour patina from the word, attempted to define propaganda by first splitting it into two categories: rational (or "good") propaganda and nonrational ("bad") propaganda. Roughly, rational propaganda is marked by a few tenets: it is *not* disguised as anything other than influential messaging (i.e., "it comes dressed in its natural clothing"), its interests are with the audience and not the self/author/rhetor, and it is attached to truth/facts of the moment (Postman, 1977). Conversely, nonrational propaganda "presents itself as something else" and seeks a habitual (oftentimes emotional) response (Postman, 1977). Oversimplification aside, the point here is that propaganda, of the rational variety, is *de rigueur* in public-facing communication. But rational propaganda can also take time; facts have to be checked, experiments and hypotheses have to be duplicated, trials have to be conducted, and results have to be analyzed before rational propaganda can be released. Propaganda, of the nonrational variety, since it needs only a polished artifice that merely *represents* fidelity, can be cobbled together rapidly, disseminated quickly, and infect public knowledge almost immediately. Huxley (1958) called this "herd poisoning" and defined it as an "active, extraverted drug. The crowd-intoxicated individual escapes from responsibility, intelligence, and morality into a kind of frantic, animal mindlessness" (V. [Propaganda under a Dictatorship], para. 6). So, while the country waited for clear, factual communication ("rational, good propaganda"), *Plandemic* poisoned the herd with self-interested and deceitful (nonrational) propaganda created to elicit a habitual, emotional response. See, the thing is, though, at some level, it spoke to us all.

There is no denying that humans are storytellers and story-seekers. As Jerome Bruner, an integral figure in the creation of narrative psychology, suggests, story and/or narrative is the process we use to create self: "No story, no self" (1999, p. 8). And if this is the case, then even devout, rational world paradigm enthusiasts contain an inherent attraction to a compelling tale. This is why, we think, *Plandemic* appeals to us all. But the true power of *Plandemic* is not that it converts believers; it is that it sows doubt. For rational paradigm stewards, the penultimate sin is ignorance—none of us want to be made a fool, especially if our lives depend on it. *Plandemic*, at the very least, causes its audiences to pause for twenty-six minutes to hear a captivating tale. That pause and perhaps the hesitancy it cultivates, at the very least, slows down our reaction time. Against a fast-moving threat like COVID-19, that hesitancy we are seeing is enough to disrupt public life as usual and destabilize coordinated action during a crisis.

CONCLUSION

The truth is, there *is* truth in *Plandemic*, just not about COVID-19. The fact that all viewers can, at some level, relate to *Plandemic*'s story means that all audiences, not just conspiracy theory fanatics, are vulnerable to its persuasive storytelling tactics. Humans crave a good story. Good stories entertain, instruct, and offer a way to escape from and navigate through everyday life. Stories connect humankind across time, place, and experience. People turn to nonfiction to learn about what is real, what is true, and what is right. People also turn to fiction to learn equally important lessons. When done well, audiences can garner valid and practical insights about the nature of truth, and life, and ethics, and beauty, even when their vehicle is characterized by falsehoods, deception, and imagination. When a story is told well, lines between fiction and nonfiction can be blurred, and in a digital environment, those distinctions become even more difficult to disentangle. We see in the case of *Plandemic* that, when in the wrong hands, the fact/fiction, truth/lie divides get blurred intentionally, manipulatively, but effectively nonetheless.

Understanding how digital media informs and transforms public understandings of public health risks amidst a crisis is essential to effectively responding to the current pandemic and to prepare for our next. That outcome may rely on our collective willingness to recognize and learn from the rhetorical prowess of manufactured disinformation rather than debunk and dismiss it. This chapter took seriously one especially powerful piece of recent disinformation that proves toxic in both content and form, the "documentary" video *Plandemic,* and evaluated it according to the value and potency of its storytelling techniques. To do so, we took seriously narrative reasoning as a valid, practical, and inclusive means for making sense of the world around us, especially during a crisis. Yes, eradicating COVID-19 will require good science, but as we have demonstrated here, it will also require telling a damn good story.

NOTES

1. Although social media blocks the original source, the authors have a copy of the original video for analysis.

REFERENCES

Andrews, T. A. (2020, May 7). Facebook and other companies are removing viral "Plandemic" conspiracy video. *The Washington Post*. Retrieved from https://www

.washingtonpost.com/technology/2020/05/07/plandemic-youtube-facebook-vimeo-remove/

Baines, A., Ittefaq, M., & Abwao, M. (2021). #Scamdemic, #Plandemic, or #Scaredemic: What Parler social media platform tells us about COVID-19 vaccine. *Vaccines*, *9*, 421. Retrieved from https://doi.org/10.3390/vaccines9050421

Brewster, J. (2020, August 19). Facebook bans users from sharing debunked "Plandemic" movie. *Forbes*. Retrieved from https://www.forbes.com/sites/jackbrewster/2020/08/18/facebook-bans-users-from-sharing-debunked-plandemic-movie/?sh=52e146e637cc

Bruner, J. (1999). Narratives of aging. *Journal of Aging Studies*, *13*, 7–9. Retrieved from https://doi.org/10.1016/S0890-4065(99)80002-4

Burke, K. (1968). *Language as symbolic action: Essays on life, literature, and method*. Berkeley: University of California Press.

Cathey, L. (2020, August 8). Timeline: Tracking Trump alongside scientific developments on hydroxychloroquine. *ABC News*. Retrieved from https://abcnews.go.com/Health/timeline-tracking-trump-alongside-scientific-developments-hydroxychloroquine/story?id=72170553

Caulley, D. N. (2008). Making qualitative research reports less boring: The techniques of writing creative nonfiction. *Qualitative Inquiry, 14* (3), 424–449. Retrieved from https://doi.org/10.1177/1077800407311961

Cheetham, J. (2021, February 15). Does yoga have a conspiracy theory problem? *BBC News*. Retrieved from https://www.bbc.com/news/world-55957298

Coles, R. (1989). *The call of stories: Teaching and the moral imagination*. Boston, MA: Houghton Mifflin.

Cook, J., van der Linden, S., Lewandowsky, S., & Ecker, U. (2020, May 15). Coronavirus, "Plandemic" and the seven traits of conspiratorial thinking. *The Conversation*. Retrieved from https://theconversation.com/coronavirus-plandemic-and-the-seven-traits-of-conspiratorial-thinking-138483

Dacombe, R. (2021, January 29). Conspiracy theories: Why are they thriving in the pandemic? *The Conversation*. Retrieved from https://theconversation.com/conspiracy-theories-why-are-they-thriving-in-the-pandemic-153657

Dickson, E. J. (2020, May 12). Judy Mikovits, disgraced doctor at the center of "Plandemic," has a bestselling book on Amazon. *Rolling Stone*. Retrieved from https://www.rollingstone.com/culture/culture-news/plandemic-judy-mikovits-plague-of-corruption-998224/

Enserink, M., & Cohen, J. (2020, May 8). Fact-checking Judy Mikovits, the controversial virologist attacking Anthony Fauci in a viral conspiracy video. *Science*. Retrieved from https://www.sciencemag.org/news/2020/05/fact-checking-judy-mikovits-controversial-virologist-attacking-anthony-fauci-viral

Fichera, A., Spencer, S. H., Gore, D., Robertson, L., & Kiely, E. (2020, May 8). The falsehoods of the "Plandemic" video. *FactCheck.org*. Retrieved from https://www.factcheck.org/2020/05/the-falsehoods-of-the-plandemic-video/

Fisher, W. R. (1984). Narration as a human communication paradigm: The case of public moral argument. *Communication Monographs*, *51*(1), 1–22. Retrieved from https://doi.org/10.1080/03637758409390180

Frenkel, S., Decker, B., & Alba, D. (2020, May 21). How the "Plandemic" movie and its falsehoods spread widely online. *The New York Times*. Retrieved from https://www.nytimes.com/2020/05/20/technology/plandemic-movie-youtube-facebook-coronavirus.html

Freytag, G. (2004). *Technique of the drama: An exposition of dramatic composition and art*. (E. J. MacEwan, Trans.). University Press of the Pacific. (Original work published in 1896).

Graff, G. M. (2020, September 10). 9/11 and the rise of the new conspiracy theorists. *The Wall Street Journal*. Retrieved from https://www.wsj.com/articles/9-11-and-the-rise-of-the-new-conspiracy-theorists-11599768458

Gutkind, L. (2006). Creative nonfiction: A movement, not a movement. *Creative Nonfiction, 29*, 6–18. Retrieved from https://creativenonfiction.org/writing/creative-nonfiction-a-movement-not-a-moment/

Gutkind, L. (2012). *You can't make this stuff up: The complete guide to writing creative nonfiction from memoir to literary journalism and everything in between*. Boston: Da Capo Press/Lifelong Books.

Hamel, L., Kirzinger, A., Muñana, C., & Brodie, M. (2020, December 15). KFF COVID-19 vaccine monitor: December 2020. *Kaiser Family Foundation*. Retrieved from https://www.kff.org/coronavirus-covid-19/report/kff-covid-19-vaccine-monitor-december-2020/

Hesse, D. (2008). Who owns creative nonfiction? In T. J. Enos, K. D. Miller, & J. McCracken (Eds.), *Beyond postprocess and postmodernism: Essays on the spaciousness of rhetoric*. 245–260. London: Taylor & Francis.

Huxley, A. (1958). *A brave new world revisited*. Retrieved from https://www.huxley.net/bnw-revisited/

Islam, M. S., Kamal, A-H. M., Kabir, A., Southern, D. L., Khan, S. H., Hasan, S. M. M., Sarkar, T., Sharmin, S., Das, S., Roy, T., Harun, M. G. D., Chughtai, A. A., Homaira, N., & Seale, H. (2021, May 12). COVID-19 vaccine rumors and conspiracy theories: The need for cognitive inoculation against misinformation to improve vaccine adherence. *PLoS One*. Retrieved from https://doi.org/10.1371/journal.pone.0251605

Konnikova, M. (2015, December 29). How stories deceive. *The New Yorker*. Retrieved from https://www.newyorker.com/science/maria-konnikova/how-stories-deceive

Lopate, P. (2013). *To show and to tell: The craft of literary nonfiction*. New York: Free Press.

Merlan, A. (2019). *Republic of lies: American conspiracy theorists and their surprising rise to power*. New York: Metropolitan Books.

Mitchell, A., Jurkowitz, M., Oliphant, J. B., & Shearer, E. (2020, June 29). Three months in, many Americans see exaggeration, conspiracy theories and partisanship in COVID-19 news. *Pew Research Center*. Retrieved from https://www.journalism.org/2020/06/29/three-months-in-many-americans-see-exaggeration-conspiracy-theories-and-partisanship-in-covid-19-news/

Nazar, S., & Pieters, T. (2021). Plandemic revisited: A product of planned disinformation amplifying the COVID-19 "infodemic." *Frontiers in Public Health*, *9*, 954. Retrieved from https://doi.org/10.3389/fpubh.2021.649930

Neuman, S. (2020, May 8). Seen "Plandemic"? We take a close look at the viral conspiracy video's claims. *NPR*. Retrieved from https://www.npr.org/2020/05/08/852451652/seen-plandemic-we-take-a-close-look-at-the-viral-conspiracy-video-s-claims\

Newton, C. (2020a, May 12). How the "Plandemic" video hoax went viral: Platforms did their best to remove a video with a harmful claim—but more than 8 million people watched it anyway. *The Verge*. Retrieved from https://www.theverge.com/2020/5/12/21254184/how-plandemic-went-viral-facebook-youtube

Newton, C. (2020b, August 19). Platforms successfully stopped a COVID conspiracy video from going viral: The trick is getting the hucksters to announce a premiere date. *The Verge*. Retrieved from https://www.theverge.com/interface/2020/8/19/21373820/plandemic-indoctornation-facebook-youtube-twitter-removal-block-covid-hoax-block

Pappas, S. (2020, May 13). Debunking the most dangerous claims of "Plandemic." *Live Science*. Retrieved from https://www.livescience.com/debunking-plandemic-coronavirus-claims.html

Picheta, R. (2019, November 18). The flat-Earth conspiracy is spreading around the globe. Does it hide a darker core? *CNN*. Retrieved from https://www.cnn.com/2019/11/16/us/flat-earth-conference-conspiracy-theories-scli-intl/index.html

Polkinghorne, D. E. (1988). *Narrative knowing and the human sciences*. Albany: State University of New York Press.

Postman, N. (1977). *Crazy talk, stupid talk: How we defeat ourselves by the way we talk and what to do about it*. New York: Doubleday.

Postman, N. (1985). *Amusing ourselves to death: Public discourse in the age of show business*. New York: Viking Penguin.

Rakedzon, T., Segev, E., Chapnik, N., Yosef, R., & Baram-Tsabari, A. (2017, August 29). Automatic jargon identifier for scientists engaging with the public and science communication educators. *PLoS One*, *12*, e0181742. Retrieved from https://doi.org/10.1371/journal.pone.0181742

Reader, R. (2021, March 24). The pernicious staying power of COVID-19's first viral disinformation campaign. *Fast Company*. Retrieved from https://www.fastcompany.com/90611781/plandemic-covid-19-viral-disinformation-campaign-staying-power

Roose, K. (2020, May 13). Get ready for a vaccine information war. *New York Times*. Retrieved from https://www.nytimes.com/2020/05/13/technology/coronavirus-vaccine-disinformation.html

Rosenblum, N. L., & Muirhead, R. (2019). *A lot of people are saying: The new conspiracism and the assault on democracy*. Princeton, NJ: Princeton University Press.

Rottenberg, J., & Perman, S. (2020, May 13). Meet the Ojai dad who made the most notorious piece of coronavirus disinformation yet. *Los Angeles Times*. Retrieved from https://www.latimes.com/entertainment-arts/movies/story/2020-05-13/plandemic-coronavirus-documentary-director-mikki-willis-mikovits

Siemaszko, C. (2017, December 5). Professor who suggested Sandy Hook massacre was hoax sues Florida Atlantic University. *NBC News*. Retrieved from https://www.nbcnews.com/news/us-news/professor-who-suggested-sandy-hook-massacre-was-hoax-sues-florida-n826646

Willis, M. (2021a, May 4). *Plandemic: The hidden agenda behind Covid-19* [Video]. Youtube.

Willis, M. (2021b). *Plandemic: Fear is the virus, truth is the cure.* New York: Skyhorse.

Wilson, J. (2020, April 7). Why Trump's media allies are turning against Fauci amid the pandemic. *The Guardian.* Retrieved from https://www.theguardian.com/us-news/2020/apr/07/fox-news-coronavirus-trump-media-allies-turn-against-fauci

Yong, A. (2020, April 29). Why the coronavirus is so confusing: A guide to making sense of a problem that is now too big for any one person to fully comprehend. *The Atlantic*. Retrieved from https://www.theatlantic.com/health/archive/2020/04/pandemic-confusing-uncertainty/610819/

Index

About the Editors and Contributors

ABOUT THE EDITORS

Shing-Ling S. Chen is professor of mass communication in the Department of Communication and Media at the University of Northern Iowa.

Nicole Allaire is associate teaching professor in the Department of English at Iowa State University.

ABOUT THE CONTRIBUTORS

Melissa L. Beall is professor of communication studies at the University of Northern Iowa. Her teaching and research interests include intercultural communication, communication theory, listening, and communication education.

Stephen D. Caldes is an assistant professor in the Department of Journalism & Public Relations at California State University, Chico. He teaches writing intensive courses on narrative nonfiction, propaganda and digital media literacy. He writes mostly about writing and writing pedagogy, but also freelances for a number of magazines where he writes about food and culture. His most recent work can be found in the *International Journal of Multidisciplinary Perspectives in Higher Education* and *Edible.*

Juliet Dee is an associate professor in the Department of Communication at the University of Delaware. She teaches courses in First Amendment law, mass media and culture, broadcast programming and television production. She has been director of the Legal Studies Program at the University of

Delaware, has been an editor of the *Free Speech Yearbook,* and is a co-author of *Mass Communication Law in a Nutshell* (2020).

Zach Justus is professor and chair of communication arts and sciences at California State University, Chico. His research is on extremist rhetoric including gun-rights and anti-immigration advocacy, and educational strategies for improving dialogue. His work can be found in *Argumentation and Advocacy* and *Communication Teacher* as well as other edited volumes and journals.

Rachel Kaplan is an assistant professor of corporate communication at Penn State University, Fayette. She is also the co-director of the Fayette LaunchBox, an on-campus business incubator. She has published numerous articles and scholarly presentations about health communication. Currently she is publishing her first book, *The Rhetoric of the Opioid Crisis*, with Lexington Books. Her areas of expertise include crisis communication, health communication, and organizational communication.

Kristjan Kikerpill is a doctoral student of sociology at the Institute of Social Studies in the University of Tartu, Estonia. His main areas of research are online deception, the mechanics of social engineering attacks, the social impact of deepfakes, and crime prevention in online environments. Recent publications include a socio-legal analysis of phishing e-mails, a critical analysis of cybercrime case law, and a criminological perspective on the role of individuals in cybercrime prevention.

Jennifer A. Malkowski is an assistant professor of communication arts and sciences at California State University, Chico. Her research and teaching lie at the intersections of public health communication, medical professionalism, and biotechnological controversy where she explores how persuasive communication influences perceptions of and responses to health risks at both the individual and collective levels. Her work appeared in *Rhetoric of Health & Medicine*, *Health Communication*, and *Journal of Medical Humanities* in addition to other journals and edited collections.

Zanetta Miller is an instructor of speech and business communication as well as a doctoral student in organizational leadership at Indiana Wesleyan University. In addition, she works as a public relations consultant and operates a senior living referral business in Northwest Indiana. Her current research focuses on leadership in the healthcare sector among female leaders in the C-Suite.

John J. Rief is assistant professor of rhetoric and debate, and director of debate in the Department of Communication Studies at Metropolitan State University of Denver. He teaches numerous courses in the areas of rhetoric in popular and public culture, argumentation and debate, and public speaking. His research interests include the history of rhetoric and intercollegiate debating in the U.S., argumentation theory, and the rhetoric of health and medicine.

Elizabeth Spradley is an assistant professor of communication studies at Stephen F. Austin State University where she also serves as program and basic course coordinator for the communication studies program. She serves on the editorial board for *The Intima: A Journal of Narrative Medicine*. Her research focuses on narrative, health, crisis/pandemic communication, and identity. Her recent work has been published in the *Journal of the Motherhood Initiative*, the *International Research Journal of Health Education*, and a number of book chapters related to narrative medicine, humor in healthcare, and pandemic communication.

R. Tyler Spradley is an associate professor of communication studies at Stephen F. Austin State University, where he was awarded the 2013–2014 and 2014–2015 Jim Towns Endowed Mentoring Professorship, and coordinates the leadership minor and certificates in risk and crisis communication and leadership. He researches high reliability organizations and teams, sociomateriality, risk and crisis communication, and human-machine communication in emergency and medical training. He has published in *The International Encyclopedia of Organizational Communication, Sage Research Methods Cases, Journal of Human Services, International Research Journal of Health Education,* and *International Research Journal of Public Health,* and he has forthcoming chapters on outdoor adventure education, religious pandemic rhetoric, pandemic theories, and working from home.

Tyler Welsh is an assistant professor of communication studies at Stephen F. Austin State University. His research focuses on rhetoric, popular culture, and publics/counterpublics. His recent work has been published in the *Journal of Popular Music and Society*, and he has presented at multiple conferences on topics related to media, sport, and symbolic influences on everyday lived experiences.

Lightning Source UK Ltd.
Milton Keynes UK
UKHW041258230622
404866UK00003B/79

9 781793 655332